Title: NEW NCLEX RN PRACTICE QUESTION BANK
Subtitle: NEXT GEN NCLEX QUESTIONS AND ANSWERS & INDEPTH EXPLANATIONS
EDITION II

Author: Anita Bhattarai
ISBN: 9798338692721

Imprint: Independently published

Copyright © 2024 by Anita Bhattarai
Cover design by Gunjan Subedi

All rights reserved. No part of this book may be reproduced or transmitted in any form or by any means, electronic or mechanical, including photocopying, recording, or any information storage and retrieval system, without permission in writing from the author, except for brief quotations in critical articles or reviews.

Disclaimer:

This book is intended to provide information and strategies for exam preparation and practice only. It is not a substitute for medical advice, nursing interventions, or treatment. The author and publisher are not responsible for any actions taken by readers based on the information presented in this book.
Every effort has been made to ensure the accuracy of the information presented in this book. However, the author and publisher do not assume any responsibility for errors or omissions. Readers are advised to seek professional advice before applying any of the strategies or information presented in this book.

The terms 'NCLEX' and 'NCSBN' (National Council of State Boards of Nursing) are not my proprietary. This book is intended to assist nursing students in preparing for the NCLEX exam by providing study material, practice questions, and test-taking strategies. The content in this book is not endorsed by or affiliated with 'NCLEX' exam or 'NCSBN'. It is important to note that passing the NCLEX exam requires a combination of knowledge, critical thinking, and test-taking skills. While this book may provide helpful resources, it is not a guarantee of passing the NCLEX exam, and it is recommended to utilize a variety of study materials and resources to prepare adequately.

First Printing: 2024

With dedication and passion so true,

There's nothing that nurses can't do!

Dedicated to all the students and nursing professionals who have put in tireless effort to realize their NCLEX RN aspirations. A heartfelt tribute goes out to my mother Padam and mother in law, Prof. Durga who instilled in me the virtues of perseverance and ethical values that have made it possible for me to guide my readers with ease.

Your unwavering support and belief in my journey have been the cornerstone of my success. This book is a testament to your love, guidance, and inspiration. May it serve as a beacon of knowledge and empowerment for all those who seek to make a difference in the noble field of nursing.

Preface:

As a nursing student myself, I recall the challenges of finding effective study materials for the NCLEX-RN exam, particularly with the recent introduction of the Next Generation NCLEX-RN format. This updated format emphasizes nursing assessments and integrates case studies that demand a distinct set of skills. My own journey to locate comprehensive and clear study resources revealed a scarcity of useful materials, often leading to confusion.

Driven by the need for a better solution, I embarked on creating a comprehensive resource tailored to nursing students preparing for the NCLEX-RN. The result of this endeavor is the 'NEW NCLEX RN PRACTICE QUESTION BANK.' This book has been meticulously revised from its first edition, addressing previous errors and aligning with the latest changes in the NCLEX format. It has been enhanced with more case studies and practical scenarios that reflect real-world nursing practice, providing a more hands-on approach to studying.

The second edition offers revised content that enhances user experience and aligns with the New Next Generation NCLEX format, addressing the errors and issues present in the first edition. This version includes a wide range of question types—like highlighting, extended multiple-choice, fill-in-the-blank, drag-and-drop, matrix, and matching pairs—accommodating the various question formats found in the exam.

This book is crafted to be an indispensable tool for nursing students and professionals seeking to deepen their knowledge and excel in the NCLEX-RN exam. While it aims to provide a thorough and practical resource, there is always room for improvement, and future editions will continue to evolve.

I hope that 'NEW NCLEX RN PRACTICE QUESTION BANK' serves as a valuable resource in your journey to becoming a nurse. Your dedication and hard work are commendable, and I am honored to contribute to your success. With this book, may you approach the NCLEX-RN exam with confidence and readiness, paving the way for a rewarding career in nursing.

ACKNOWLEDGMENTS

Many of my friends and students achieved success on their first attempts at the NCLEX, igniting a ripple of accomplishment among my professional circles. Witnessing their triumphs prompted them to seek my guidance. Their victories, coupled with their gratitude for my ability to simplify complex topics and illustrate practical scenarios drawn from my decade-long nursing experience and teaching, served as the impetus behind my decision to craft a foundational support guide for conquering the NCLEX with ease.

Initially conceived as a tool for my friends, this guidebook gradually evolved into a global resource, offering a spectrum of strategies, Question formats, and illustrative examples aimed at bolstering confidence for NCLEX preparation.

I extend heartfelt appreciation to all my friends whose achievements inspired me to publish this book. A special acknowledgment goes to my mother-in-law, Prof. Durga, and my husband, Gunjan, for their steadfast encouragement and unwavering support throughout this journey.

"Humanity and love exist! Last but not least, I would also like to thank Monica Rego (whom I respectfully and loving call 'Bonus Mom') who has been helping with everything recently, making my nursing journey easier and allowing me the interest and courage to embark on writing this vast book!"

Anita B.

Table of Contents

FEELING LUCKY ? 8
HOW TO USE THIS BOOK ? 9
PREPARATION TIPS 11
Reducing exam stress 11
Preparing for the NCLEX: The Importance of Habit 12
Keep a track of your time 13
Maximizing Your Study Time for Exam Success 13
Regularly Practice Next Generation NClex-RN related Questions-Answers 15
Pamper Yourself 16

BREAKDOWN OF EXAM CONTENT 17
Safe and Effective Care Environment 17
Health Promotion and Maintenance 18
Psychosocial Integrity 18
Physiological Integrity 18

ALL ABOUT NEXT/NEW GENERATION NCLEX (NGN) 19
Delivery Method 20
How CAT Works: 20
Pass/Fail Determination 20
Some Basic Tips to follow in solving the questions. 24
Prioritization words 26
Take care of closed-ended Words 28
Take care of Prioritization 30
Situations Requiring Immediate or Urgent Prioritization 30
Situations Requiring Intermediate Priority 30
Situations Requiring Low Priority 30
Finding options with urgent priority with keywords 32
When to choose the option 'Call the health care provider'? 32
Prioritizing with the focus or strategic words and statements 33
Prioritizing based on any special steps in nursing procedure which you must not escape. 35
Prioritizing based on ABC 36
Prioritizing based on CABC 36
Prioritizing based on Maslow's hierarchy of needs. 38
Prioritization with Emergency Department Triage 40
Emergent or Highest Priority Clients (Red Zone) 40
Urgent or Intermediate Priority (Yellow Zone) 40
Non-urgent or Least Priority (Green Zone) 40
Eliminating similar options 41

TYPES OF QUESTION FORMAT IN NEXT GENERATION NCLEX 43
Case Study Question : Introduction 44
What do these cognitive skills entail? 45
Effective Strategies for Handling Case Studies 45
Extended Multiple options or Multiple Answer Questions 47
Extended Drag and Drop Questions 50
Cloze Type Questions 52
Matrix/ Grid Type Questions 54
Highlighting 56
Other Question Types for Standalone Questions 57

- Multiple Choice Question 57
- Figure Questions 57
- Chart/Table Type Questions 59
- Fill in the blanks type question 61
- Multiple options/Response Questions 64

PART I: NCLEX MASTERY: ESSENTIAL CATEGORIES AND KEY FOCUS AREAS FOR SUCCESS 65

- Ethical / Legal aspects/ Professional Standards in Nursing 65
- Positioning of the patient 74
- Total Parenteral Nutrition 78
- Blood and Blood Products 81
- Blood Components 87
- Medication Administration 90
- Administration of Blood Products 92
- Managing Anaphylactic reactions 95
- Practice Session 97
- Emergency Department Triage 106
- IV Solutions 119
- Catheters and Tubing 123
- Infection Control 129
- Theories of Growth and Development 136
- Practice Session 137
- Preoperative Care 139
- Burn and Management 143
- Endocrine System 148
- Nursing therapies 158
- Practice Session- 159
- Pediatric Nursing 162
- Gerontology /Geriatric Nursing 166
- Nervous System/ Diseases 171
- Seizure 177
- Parkinson's Disease 179
- Musculo-Skeletal System /Drugs 181
- Gout and Management 181
- Osteoarthritis 184
- Rheumatoid arthritis 186
- Renal and Urinary System 188
- Obstetrics and Gynaecology 190
- Reproductive System 190
- Eyes and Ears 195
- Cardiovascular System/circulatory disorders 200
- Gastrointestinal disorders 203

PART II: PHARMACOLOGICAL INTERVENTIONS 205

- Antibiotics: Introduction and classification 205
- NSAIDS AND OPOIDS: Introduction and classification 210
- Antidepressants and anti-anxiety 214
- Anticoagulants and Antiplatelet 221
- Cardiovascular medication 225
- Antiarrhythmics 228
- Cardiovascular drugs-digoxin 231
- Antidiabetic medication 233
- Psychotropic Medications 239

- Antiemetics and Gastrointestinal drugs 242
- Antihypertensives 246
- Diuretics 250
- Tuberculosis Medications 254
- Integumentary system / Drugs 257
- Antifungal Medications... 260
- Narcotic Antagonists 265
- Anticancer 268
- Palliative Care Principles.. 272

FURTHER READING : RECOMMENDED RESOURCES 276

Feeling Lucky ?

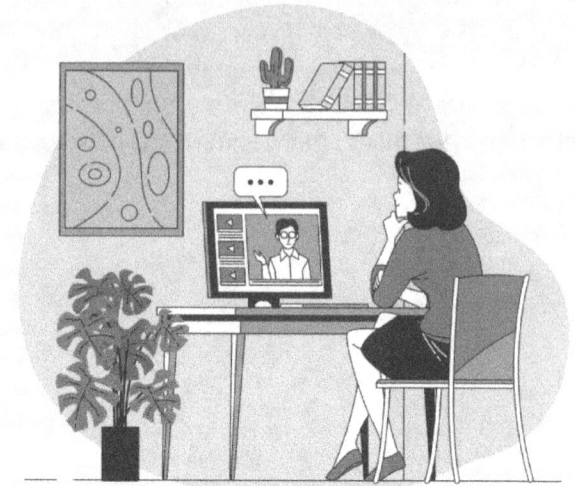

00:00:00:00
DAYS HOURS MINUTES SECONDS

100 STUDENTS SELECTED EACH MONTH !
JOIN THE FREE FASTTRACK NCLEX-RN CRASH COURSE BEFORE THE LINK EXPIRES...
IT'S 100% FREE
SCROLL DOWN FOR DETAILS !!!

First name

Email

Let's Get Started

Attention all nursing students!

Every month, we randomly select 100 students to participate in our free fast track NCLEX RN practice course. This could be your chance to join and take the first step towards achieving your dream of becoming a registered nurse. Our course is tailored to provide you with comprehensive and effective practice resources that will help you build the necessary knowledge and skills to excel in your exam. Our expertly crafted study materials and practice tests will set you on the path to success. Don't miss out on this opportunity, sign up now and start your journey to becoming a registered nurse!

LINK- https://www.nclexmentors.com/freenclexcrashcourse

For other free resources, join us,

Youtube: https://www.youtube.com/@nextgenerationnclexmentors

Facebook (New Page):

https://www.facebook.com/groups/2295458660638596

How to use this book ?

Welcome to the "How to Use This Book" section of this nursing textbook. This section will guide you through the different sections of the book and help you understand how to use each section effectively.

This book is organized in a way that allows readers to navigate efficiently through a wide range of topics related to NCLEX RN exam preparation. The structure begins with general advice on exam readiness, such as preparation tips and stress management, before gradually diving into more detailed content. To start using the book, you might first want to focus on the initial sections that provide strategies for creating effective study habits and maximizing study time. These parts help lay the foundation for tackling more complex material, ensuring you have the right mindset and plan in place before diving into specific nursing topics.

As you progress, the book organizes its core content around critical exam areas like patient care environments, health promotion, and prioritization techniques. The breakdown of these sections makes it easier to concentrate on particular aspects of the NCLEX, allowing you to focus on the topics that may need more attention. For example, there are comprehensive sections on handling emergency triage, prioritizing based on Maslow's Hierarchy of Needs, and eliminating incorrect answers. Each segment presents practical examples and strategies, guiding you in tackling exam questions effectively.

The next section of the book emphasize practice and application, especially regarding question formats that you'll likely encounter in the NCLEX. It covers various question types such as multiple choice, drag-and-drop, and matrix/grid-type questions, which mirror the Next Generation NCLEX.

Part I of the book, titled "NCLEX Mastery: Essential Categories and Key Focus Areas for Success," delves into the most critical areas of nursing knowledge that the NCLEX tests. It is designed to help students solidify their grasp of core nursing concepts. This section covers important topics like ethical/legal aspects of nursing, patient positioning, and the administration of medications, such as blood products and nutritional therapies. It also addresses practical areas like managing anaphylactic reactions, infection control, and emergency department triage, all of which are vital for real-world nursing practice. Part I is structured to ensure that readers can not only memorize key information but also understand how to apply it in clinical situations, enhancing both test performance and practical nursing competence.

Part II, "Pharmacological Interventions," takes a deep dive into drug classifications, mechanisms, and the nursing responsibilities associated with medication administration. This section is crucial for mastering pharmacology, which is often a challenging aspect of the NCLEX. It covers various types of medications, from antibiotics and NSAIDs to psychotropic drugs and cardiovascular medications. The detailed explanations of drug interactions, side effects, and therapeutic uses help readers build confidence in handling pharmacological questions. In addition, the section provides focused content on specialized drugs, such as anticancer agents and antifungal medications, ensuring that you have a broad and in-depth understanding of pharmacological interventions as they apply to nursing care.

To make the most of this section, we recommend that you start by reading the introduction to each topic, which provides a brief overview of the key concepts. Then, move on to the strategy section, which will give you different approaches to solving nursing problems related to that topic. After that, complete the practice section and case study to apply the strategies you've learned and test your understanding.

Some key areas can be discovered with diagrams they come up with:

Strategy Section: This section covers the strategies that can be applied to solve the problem in the practice section. Whenever you reach following discover that you have reached the strategy section which is usually first section of the topic.

Practice Section: The practice section/session contains practice questions, case studies and answers with explanation of each options. This helps you to understand how you may be tempted to select a wrong option and how to avoid that.

NGN Case Study Section: This section contains a case study scenario which may contain history of disease, nurse's notes, physician's orders, lab values etc. A single case study contains 6 different questions related to case study.

Preparation TIPs

Reducing exam stress

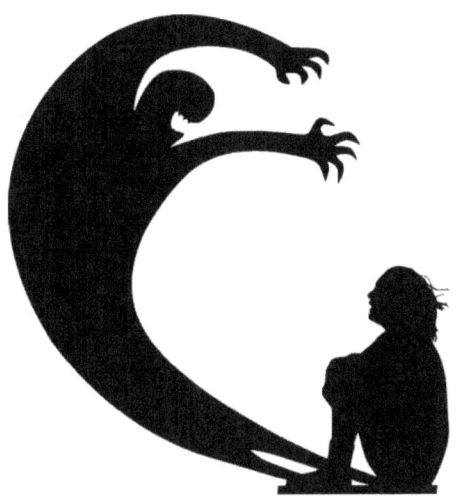

Test anxiety is a well-known phenomenon that is experienced by countless students, especially those who are preparing for or taking the NCLEX examination. In this chapter, we will delve into the possible causes of test anxiety and explore effective strategies for reducing or eliminating them. Whether you're a nursing student still in school or a seasoned professional preparing for the NCLEX, this guide will equip you with the tools to perform your best on test day.

As you may already know, test anxiety can manifest in a variety of physical and emotional symptoms. For example, you may experience dizziness, stomach acidity, abdominal pain, headache, vomiting, restlessness, and other unpleasant sensations when faced with a challenging exam. This is especially true for the NCLEX, which demands a high level of cognitive engagement and sustained attention. Knowing how to manage these symptoms is crucial for success on the exam.

It's not uncommon for even the most diligent and well-prepared students to feel overwhelmed or "blank out" during an exam. This can be a particularly frustrating experience, especially if you've put in hours of study and practice. However, it's important to recognize that these are all symptoms of test anxiety and can be addressed with the right approach.

Throughout this chapter, we will explore various techniques for managing test anxiety and improving your performance on the NCLEX. From mindfulness exercises to relaxation techniques, we will cover a range of strategies that can help you stay calm, focused, and confident on test day. So whether you're a first-time test taker or a seasoned pro, this guide has something for everyone. With the right mindset and tools, you can overcome test anxiety and perform your best on the NCLEX exam.

Let's first start with the preparation phase and how to reduce exam anxiety in this phase.

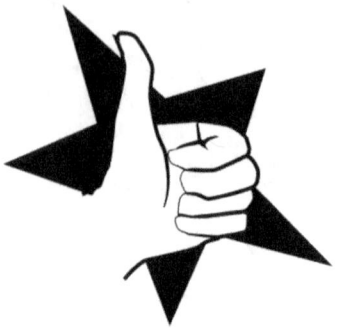

Preparing for the NCLEX: The Importance of Habit

Creating a study plan is essential for success in the NCLEX RN exam. If you haven't established one yet, now is the ideal time to start. A well-structured study plan will not only guide your preparation but also help you manage your time effectively. It's crucial to eliminate distractions, particularly your cell phone, during study hours. By committing to a distraction-free environment, you can enhance your focus, retain information better, and ultimately maximize your productivity during each session.

When designing your study plan, allocate specific time slots for studying, varying from 30 minutes to 2 hours based on your preference and capacity for concentration. Long, unbroken study periods can lead to fatigue, so it's important to avoid burnout. Consider incorporating the Pomodoro technique into your routine: study intensely for 25 minutes, then take a 5-minute break. This method can significantly improve your concentration and efficiency, allowing your brain to recharge. Additionally, set daily goals for practice questions and review sessions. Tracking your progress will not only keep you motivated but also help you identify areas that need more attention.

Choosing the right environment is also a key factor in your study success. Find a quiet, well-ventilated space that you can consistently use for your study sessions. A familiar environment will help create a productive atmosphere, minimizing the potential for distractions. Furthermore, consider waking up early to study; the mornings often provide a calm and peaceful setting that can enhance focus and productivity. By following these strategies—developing a solid study plan, committing to focused study sessions, and creating a conducive study environment—you can pave the way for success in the NCLEX exam and achieve your goal of becoming a registered nurse.

Keep a track of your time

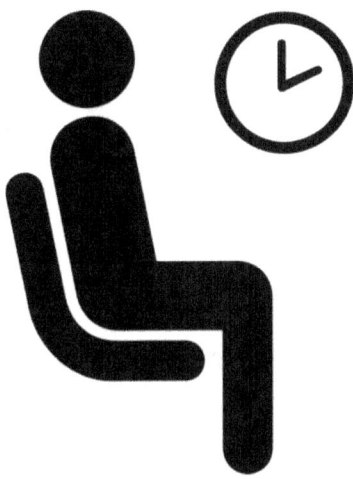

Maximizing Your Study Time for Exam Success

Optimizing your study time is essential for enhancing your chances of success in any course or exam. One of the key strategies to save time involves utilizing available resources effectively. For instance, as a student in my course, you can access audio lectures found in the resources section. By downloading these audio files after watching the video lectures, you can listen to them during commutes or while relaxing. This approach allows you to engage with the material in a more flexible manner, ensuring you stay up-to-date without sacrificing valuable time.

Additionally, I have created a free fast-track NCLEX RN practice course, which offers a limited number of free course login passes for students. This course provides a great opportunity to sharpen your skills and test your knowledge as you prepare for the exam. You can access the link here: https://rb.gy/7izw6d. This resource can complement your studies, offering practice materials that are crucial for your success.

Keeping track of your time is equally important. Implementing time management tools like ASANA or even simple notebooks can help you monitor your study habits effectively. By setting daily, weekly, and monthly goals, and diligently tracking your progress, you can manage your time better and maintain focus on your studies. As the exam date approaches, it's critical to minimize distractions from social media, entertainment, or travel. This is a time for deep concentration and commitment to your studies. If you're looking for additional tips on how to stay focused and avoid distractions, numerous online resources can guide you, including articles that provide effective strategies for maintaining your concentration. By employing these techniques and leveraging valuable resources, you can optimize your study time and significantly enhance your chances of achieving success in your exams.

Prepare Yourself

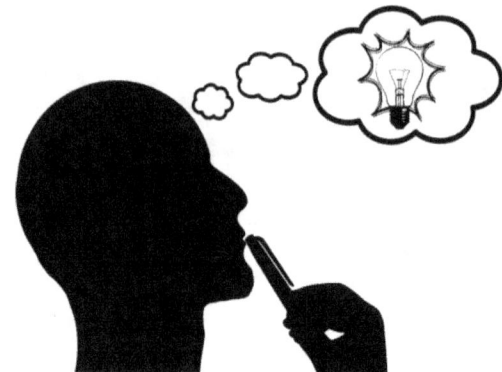

Preparing for an exam goes beyond simply gaining knowledge; it also involves nurturing your body and mind. Maintaining a healthy lifestyle during your study period is crucial. This includes regular exercise, a balanced diet, sufficient sleep, and effective relaxation techniques. By prioritizing your physical and mental well-being, you'll enhance your ability to concentrate and study efficiently, which will ultimately lead to improved performance on exam day.

A key aspect of getting ready for the NCLEX exam is becoming familiar with the various question formats you may encounter. This can include scenarios involving positive and negative events, prioritization challenges, communication-based questions, and more. To aid in your preparation, our course features a comprehensive series of video lectures designed specifically for these question types. It's vital to engage with these materials well in advance of the exam to ensure you're prepared for the different formats you'll face on test day.

Whether you choose to study independently or in a group largely depends on your personal preferences. Some students thrive when studying alone, while others benefit from collaborative learning. However, it's important to make the most of your group study sessions by focusing on relevant topics and avoiding time-wasting discussions. Use this time effectively to review key concepts and support one another in clarifying any uncertainties.

Our course offers a dedicated Facebook group for all students, which serves as an invaluable resource for staying informed about important announcements, sharing practice questions, and discussing relevant topics. Joining this group and actively engaging in discussions is essential, especially when peers pose questions that can benefit the entire community.

When preparing for the NCLEX exam, remember that sometimes less is more. With a plethora of books and resources available, it can be easy to feel overwhelmed. We recommend focusing on one or two high-quality textbooks along with a couple of practice question resources. We personally suggest UWorld and Saunders, although there are many other excellent options out there. Finding the right balance between having sufficient study materials and avoiding information overload is key. To get started, here's a link to a free crash course: https://www.nclexmentors.com/freenclexcrashcourse

Enhancing Knowledge Understanding

Engaging in regular practice with a question bank allows students to pinpoint their knowledge gaps. This focused approach helps them identify specific subjects where improvement is needed, enabling them to concentrate their study efforts on those areas. By addressing these weaknesses, students enhance their likelihood of achieving success on their exams.

Acquaintance with Exam Structure

The Next Generation NCLEX RN exam introduces various question formats, such as matrix, highlighting, extended drag and drop, matching, and more. Regularly practicing with a question bank familiarizes students with these diverse question styles. This familiarity not only boosts their confidence but also ensures they feel well-prepared when facing the exam.

Developing Time Management Skills

Time management is crucial for success on the NCLEX RN exam, which is strictly timed. By practicing with a question bank, students can better gauge how much time they need to answer each question. This experience helps them improve their pacing, enabling them to respond to questions both quickly and accurately.

Building Self-Confidence

Frequent practice with a question bank contributes to a student's self-confidence regarding their knowledge and skills. Regularly tackling practice questions reinforces their understanding and helps alleviate anxiety as exam day approaches. This increased confidence can significantly impact their overall performance.

Assessing Strengths and Weaknesses

Through consistent practice with a question bank, students can gain valuable insights into their strengths and weaknesses. This awareness allows them to target areas that require additional focus while also leveraging their strengths. By strategically approaching their studies, they can enhance their chances of success on the exam.

Pamper Yourself

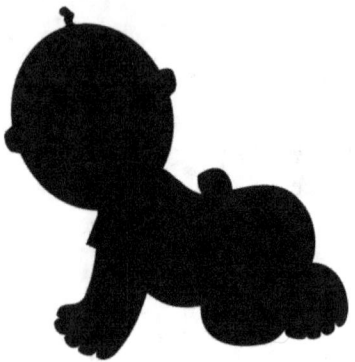

Taking Care of Yourself: Finding Balance in Your Studies

Maintaining a healthy balance between study and relaxation is vital, especially when preparing for the NCLEX. Instead of wasting hours on social media or watching endless movies, consider engaging in activities that truly refresh you. Going for a stroll in the park or having meaningful conversations with friends and family can significantly reduce stress, helping you return to your studies with renewed energy and focus.

Incorporating relaxation techniques into your routine can also be beneficial. Simple practices like deep breathing and mindfulness meditation can help calm your mind and enhance concentration. By taking a few moments each day to focus on relaxation, you can alleviate anxiety and create a more conducive environment for studying.

As you prepare for the NCLEX, remember to set realistic expectations for yourself. It's not necessary to master every single topic; focus on doing your best and answering questions thoughtfully. Visualizing your success, such as imagining yourself as an RN, can serve as a powerful motivator. Ultimately, be gentle with yourself; passing the NCLEX is just one step in your journey, and many successful nurses have faced similar challenges along the way. Keep pushing forward!

Breakdown of Exam Content

Category/Subcategory	Percentage Range
Safe and Effective Care Environment	15–21%
- Management of Care	10–16%
- Safety and Infection Control	15–21%
Health Promotion and Maintenance	6–12%
Psychosocial Integrity	6–12%
Physiological Integrity	
- Basic Care and Comfort	6–12%
- Pharmacological and Parenteral Therapies	13–19%
- Reduction of Risk Potential	9–15%
- Physiological Adaptation	11–17%

Source: nclex.com/test-plans.page

Safe and Effective Care Environment

The Safe and Effective Care Environment category focuses on ensuring the overall safety and management of healthcare, which includes crucial aspects like infection control. It is divided into two main subcategories: Management of Care, which accounts for 10–16%, and Safety and Infection Control, representing 15–21%. The primary goal is to enhance client outcomes by improving the care delivery setting, thereby safeguarding both clients and healthcare personnel. Key responsibilities in this area include integrating advance directives into care plans, delegating and supervising care, and organizing workloads for optimal time management. Nurses are expected to advocate for cost-effective care, regularly update client care plans, and educate clients and staff on their rights and responsibilities. Effective collaboration with multidisciplinary teams, conflict management, and maintaining client confidentiality are essential components. Additionally, this category encompasses accurate documentation, safe handling of admissions, transfers, and discharges, prioritizing care based on acuity, and addressing ethical dilemmas. Verifying client education and consent, implementing healthcare provider orders, utilizing resources for quality care, and participating in performance improvement projects are also vital responsibilities.

Health Promotion and Maintenance

The Health Promotion and Maintenance category emphasizes strategies and practices aimed at promoting health and preventing disease, covering 6–12% of client needs. Nurses play a crucial role in applying principles of growth and development to detect and address health issues early, as well as implementing strategies for optimal health across all life stages—from newborns to older adults. This includes providing education and care related to prenatal and post-partum needs. Nurses assess clients for health risks, learning readiness, and barriers to care, while also planning community health education initiatives and offering preventive advice. They perform targeted screenings, manage communication barriers, and ensure comprehensive health assessments to support effective home care management.

Psychosocial Integrity

The Psychosocial Integrity category focuses on the psychological and social aspects of care, constituting 6–12% of client needs. It aims to promote emotional, mental, and social well-being, especially for clients undergoing stressful experiences or dealing with acute or chronic mental health conditions. Nurses are responsible for assessing clients for potential abuse or neglect, implementing behavioral management techniques, and addressing substance abuse issues. They support clients through life transitions, evaluate risks of violence, and incorporate cultural practices into care plans. Furthermore, nurses provide end-of-life care, assess client support systems, and address grief and loss. Managing psychosocial health challenges such as addiction and depression involves recognizing non-verbal stress cues, utilizing therapeutic communication, and fostering a supportive therapeutic environment.

Physiological Integrity

Physiological Integrity is a broad category divided into four subcategories: Basic Care and Comfort (6–12%), Pharmacological and Parenteral Therapies (13–19%), Reduction of Risk Potential (9–15%), and Physiological Adaptation (11–17%). This area emphasizes promoting physical health through various nursing interventions, including providing fundamental care and comfort, assisting with daily activities, managing bowel and bladder issues, and conducting skin assessments. Nurses must also address pain management, nutritional needs, and grief while supporting clients through procedures such as post-mortem care. In Pharmacological and Parenteral Therapies, nurses are responsible for the safe administration of medications, which involves calculating dosages, educating clients, monitoring responses, and participating in medication reconciliation. Reduction of Risk Potential focuses on minimizing complications from existing conditions or treatments, requiring tasks such as monitoring vital signs, performing diagnostic tests, and ensuring client safety during procedures. Lastly, Physiological Adaptation involves managing care for clients with acute, chronic, or life-threatening conditions, assisting with invasive procedures, monitoring vital equipment, providing postoperative care, and addressing issues like fluid imbalances and impaired ventilation.

Source: nclex.com/test-plans.page

All about Next/New Generation NCLEX (NGN)

The Next Generation NCLEX (NGN) started on April 1, 2023.

Reason for Changes: The NCSBN conducted a survey to determine the knowledge and skills required for nursing practice and identified the need for better clinical judgment among nurses. To address this, the NGN includes new question formats designed to measure candidates' clinical judgment.

Content to be Studied: The core content to be studied remains the same as the previous NCLEX. Therefore, the books and materials you are currently using will still be helpful for preparing for the NGN.

Scoring Method:

Partial Credit: In the new format, candidates can receive partial credit for 'select all that apply' questions if they choose some correct options.

0/1 Rule: For certain question types, such as those requiring paired information, both parts must be correct to receive credit. If one part is wrong, the question will not be scored. For questions that ask for the order of procedures, the entire order must be correct.

Similarities with Old Exam:

Exam Duration: Candidates will have five hours to complete the exam, the same as the current NCLEX.

Performance Report: The performance report format will be similar to the current NCLEX, with the addition of a score for clinical judgment. This score will be broken down into six categories: Recognize cues, Analyze cues, Prioritize hypotheses, Generate solutions, Take actions, and Evaluate outcomes.

Delivery Method: The exam will continue to be a Computerized Adaptive Test (CAT), where the difficulty and length of questions and exam duration depend on the candidate's performance.Exam Length

The NCLEX-RN® exam consists of a minimum of 85 questions, including 70 scored items and 15 pretest items. Out of the scored questions, 52 are stand-alone items and 18 are related to clinical judgment case studies. The exam can have up to 150 questions, with a maximum of 135 scored items and 15 pretest items. Case studies comprise six questions each, evaluating various clinical judgment skills across different content areas. The total number of questions and time spent varies with each candidate's responses. To effectively manage time, candidates should aim to spend about one to two minutes per question. The length of the exam does not influence the final result, as passing or failing is determined separately from the number of questions answered.

Delivery Method

The assessment will utilize a Computerized Adaptive Test (CAT) format. This approach tailors the difficulty level and length of questions, as well as the overall exam duration, to each candidate's performance. Unlike traditional examinations, where every test-taker answers the same questions, CAT adapts to provide a more precise measurement of an individual's knowledge. In conventional tests, high-achieving candidates may find themselves answering overly simplistic questions, while those with lower ability levels might struggle with more challenging ones.

How CAT Works:

Customized Questions: The CAT system selects questions from a diverse database aligned with the exam requirements, offering a balanced representation of topics. For clinical judgment assessments, it incorporates both case studies and standalone questions based on the exam's length.

Targeted Difficulty: The technology estimates each candidate's performance and chooses questions that present a roughly 50% likelihood of correct answers. This targeted approach enhances the accuracy of knowledge assessment.

Unique Questions: Candidates taking the exam multiple times will not encounter repeated questions, maintaining the test's integrity and relevance.

Pass/Fail Determination

The results of the NCLEX exam are determined by one of three primary methods:

95% Confidence Interval Rule: This is the most common approach. The examination concludes when the system is 95% confident that a candidate's performance is clearly above or below the passing standard.

Maximum-Length Exam: For candidates whose abilities are close to the passing benchmark, the exam continues until the maximum question limit is reached. At this stage, the confidence interval is disregarded, and the final decision relies solely on the candidate's overall performance:

If the final assessment meets or exceeds the passing standard, the candidate passes.

If it falls short, the candidate fails.

Run-Out-of-Time Rule (R.O.O.T.): If a candidate runs out of time without a conclusive assessment, different rules apply:

Candidates who have not completed the minimum required number of questions will automatically fail.

For those who have met the minimum, the final outcome is based on the overall ability estimate derived from their completed answers. A score that meets or surpasses the passing standard results in a pass; otherwise, the candidate fails.

Agrima's Journey to the NCLEX RN Exam

Meet Agrima, a passionate nurse from overseas, eager to practice as a registered nurse in the United States. Her path to realizing this ambition involved several crucial steps, including passing the NCLEX and completing the CGFNS credentialing process. Here's a glimpse into how Agrima transformed her dream into reality.

Step 1: A New Beginning

Agrima's American dream started with the formidable challenge of passing the NCLEX, the licensing exam for nurses in the U.S. Understanding the necessity of rigorous preparation, she devised a structured study plan months ahead of time. Inspired by the success stories of friends who had succeeded through self-study, Agrima committed to consistent practice. She explored various study materials and question banks, ultimately choosing resources that were high-quality yet cost-effective.

Key Insights:

Prioritize Quality: Agrima focused on study guides and question banks known for their accuracy and relevance, avoiding overly expensive or low-value options.

Diverse Question Banks: She selected question banks that provided extensive coverage and clear explanations, enhancing her understanding of the material.

Organized Study Guides: Choosing well-structured study guides helped streamline her preparation.

Current Review Materials: Agrima opted for resources that were regularly updated to reflect the latest NCLEX standards.

With careful selection of her study materials, Agrima felt prepared and confident for her upcoming exam.

Step 2: The CGFNS Process

Before registering for the NCLEX, Agrima needed to have her nursing credentials evaluated by the Commission on Graduates of Foreign Nursing Schools (CGFNS). Here's how she navigated this process:

Application: Agrima filled out the online application for the CGFNS Credentials Evaluation Service (CES), providing detailed information about her nursing education.

Document Collection: She gathered essential documents, including her transcript, diplomas, nursing license from her home country, and passport.

Evaluation: CGFNS reviewed her documents to ensure her education met U.S. standards.

Credential Report: After evaluation, CGFNS issued a report confirming whether her education was equivalent to a U.S. Bachelor's degree.

With the CGFNS report in hand, Agrima was ready to proceed with her NCLEX application.

Step 3: Selecting a State

Agrima needed to choose a state Board of Nursing (BON) for her application, as requirements varied by state. She conducted thorough research and reached out to IPASS Processing for a free assessment of her documents. She discovered that some states issued nursing licenses immediately after passing the NCLEX, simplifying her process.

Step 4: Applying for Licensure

Agrima began her application for licensure by examination at least six months before her planned exam date to ensure a smooth process. She carefully completed the online application for her chosen state and paid the required fee.

Tip: Knowing her application would be valid for only one year, Agrima was diligent about meeting all requirements within that timeframe.

Step 5: Staying on Track

While waiting for her BON approval, Agrima maintained her study routine. With the approval process taking about 6-8 months, she used this time wisely to keep her skills sharp for the NCLEX.

Step 6: Registering for the NCLEX

Once Agrima received her Authorization to Test (ATT) from the BON, she registered for the NCLEX through Pearson VUE. She ensured that her registration details matched her identification exactly to avoid complications.

Tip: If she needed to register by phone, she knew to contact Pearson VUE candidate services for assistance.

Step 7: Scheduling the Exam

With her ATT secured, Agrima scheduled her NCLEX exam, carefully selecting a convenient date and location.

Tip: She made sure to book her appointment early, avoiding the last-minute rush that could lead to extra fees or complications.

Step 8: Exam Day

On the day of the exam, Agrima arrived at the testing center early. Having visited the location prior, she felt confident and prepared as she tackled the test.

Step 9: Awaiting Results

Agrima eagerly anticipated her results, which arrived within 48 hours. She checked her state BON's website and was overjoyed to see her license posted online, marking a significant milestone in her journey.

Step 10: Understanding the Scoring Process

Agrima understood that the NCLEX scoring involved two steps for quality assurance: her exam was scored at the test center and then again by Pearson VUE. Official results would be sent via her nursing regulatory body (NRB) within six weeks.

She refrained from contacting NCSBN or Pearson VUE for updates, choosing to wait patiently for her official results.

Step 11: Checking for Quick Results

Agrima explored whether her NRB offered a Quick Results service and followed the necessary steps to access her scores online. She also considered the Pearson VUE trick, an unofficial method to gauge her results, but she remained aware that only the NRB's results were definitive.

Quick Tip: Agrima recognized that unofficial results could not replace the official ones, which were crucial for her licensing.

Step 12: Reviewing the Candidate Performance Report

If the results were not what she hoped for, Agrima would receive a Candidate Performance Report (CPR) detailing her performance strengths and weaknesses. This feedback would guide her preparation for a retake, if necessary.

Step 13: Planning for a Possible Retake

Should Agrima need to retake the exam, she was prepared. According to NCSBN policy, candidates must wait at least 45 days before retaking the NCLEX and can attempt it up to eight times a year. She planned to review her CPR carefully to refine her study strategies, ensuring she was ready for her next attempt.

Agrima's journey was a testament to her dedication and resilience, proving that with the right preparation and mindset, dreams can indeed become reality.

Some Basic Tips to follow in solving the questions.

1. Grasp the Scenario: Understand the situation or context described in the question.

2. Spot Key Terms: Identify crucial words like "immediate," "initial," "priority," "best," "follow-up," or "further teaching" to determine what the question is asking.

3. Review All Options: For multiple-choice, multiple-response, or prioritization questions, read every option thoroughly before making a decision.

4. Eliminate Incorrect Choices: Use the process of elimination to narrow down your options. After eliminating the wrong ones, re-read the question to confirm your final answer.

5. Visualize the Situation: Picture the clinical scenario to identify any abnormalities in the data provided.

6. Determine the Nature of the Question: Check if the question is asking about a positive or negative event.

7. Eliminate Similar Options: Remove options that are alike or redundant.

8. Look for Broad Options: Identify if there is an umbrella option that covers other choices, which might be the correct answer.

9. Identify Absolute Terms: Be cautious of options with closed-ended words; they are often incorrect.

10. Use Prioritization Frameworks: Apply the ABCs (Airway, Breathing, Circulation), Maslow's Hierarchy of Needs, and the Nursing Process to prioritize actions.

11. Apply Therapeutic Communication: Focus on the client's thoughts, feelings, concerns, anxieties, and fears for communication questions.

12. Delegate Appropriately: Match the client's needs with the scope of practice of the healthcare provider.

Example

A patient develops a hemolytic transfusion reaction after receiving mismatched blood, presenting with fever, chills, and back pain.

Multiple-Choice Question

Question: What are the immediate nursing interventions for a patient experiencing a hemolytic transfusion reaction?

1. Stop the transfusion immediately.
2. Administer antihistamines.
3. Notify the healthcare provider.
4. Continue the transfusion at a slower rate.
5. Monitor vital signs closely.

Correct Answers: 1 and 3

Strategy to Solve the Problem

Understand the Question Context: Recognize that the question is about immediate nursing interventions for a hemolytic transfusion reaction. This sets the stage for identifying the urgency and type of actions required.

Identify Key Words: Focus on terms like "immediate nursing interventions" and "hemolytic transfusion reaction." These words indicate that the actions needed are urgent and specific to the reaction.

Read All Options Carefully: Review each option to determine its relevance to the scenario. This ensures that no potential correct answer is overlooked.

Use Elimination Process: Discard options that are not appropriate for immediate intervention. For example, continuing the transfusion at a slower rate is not suitable in this context.

Visualize the Scenario: Imagine the clinical situation and the urgency of the patient's condition. This helps in understanding the critical nature of the interventions required.

Determine Question Type: Recognize that the question is asking for immediate actions. This helps in prioritizing the options that need to be taken first.

Eliminate Similar Options: Remove options that are redundant or less critical. For instance, monitoring vital signs is important but not the first immediate action.

Look for broad Options: Identify options that broadly address the immediate needs. Stopping the transfusion immediately is a broad action that addresses the primary issue.

Explanation of Each Option

1. **Stop the transfusion immediately:** Correct. This is the first and most critical step to prevent further hemolysis.

2. **Administer antihistamines**: **Incorrect**. Antihistamines are not the primary intervention for hemolytic reactions; they are more relevant for allergic reactions.

3. **Notify the healthcare provider**: **Correct**. Prompt communication with the healthcare provider is essential for further management.

4. **Continue the transfusion at a slower rate**: **Incorrect**. Continuing the transfusion, even at a slower rate, can worsen the reaction.

5. **Monitor vital signs closely**: **Incorrect**. While monitoring is important, it is not the immediate action needed to stop the reaction.

Prioritization words

When prioritizing nursing care, certain words and phrases signal the need for immediate attention. These include:

- First
- Initial
- Early
- Best
- Next
- Most important
- Highest priority
- Vital
- Primary

Mr. Smith, a 58-year-old patient, has been managing Type 2 diabetes for the past 10 years. He visits the clinic for a routine check-up and discusses his recent blood sugar levels and lifestyle habits with the nurse. Mr. Smith mentions that he has been experiencing frequent episodes of hyperglycemia, especially after meals. He also reports feeling fatigued and has noticed some weight gain over the past few months. His current medications include metformin and insulin.

Which of the following statements made by the nurse indicates correct diabetes management advice? (Select two correct answers)

"You should first monitor your blood sugar levels before and after meals to understand how different foods affect your glucose levels."

"It's most important to avoid all carbohydrates to keep your blood sugar levels stable."

"Regular physical activity can initially help improve your insulin sensitivity and manage your weight."

"You should only take your insulin if your blood sugar levels are above 200 mg/dL."

"Skipping meals can help you avoid high blood sugar levels."

Explanation:

Correct: "You should first monitor your blood sugar levels before and after meals to understand how different foods affect your glucose levels."

Monitoring blood sugar levels before and after meals helps patients understand the impact of different foods on their glucose levels, allowing for better management of their diet and medication.

Incorrect: "It's most important to avoid all carbohydrates to keep your blood sugar levels stable."

While managing carbohydrate intake is crucial, completely avoiding all carbohydrates is not recommended. Carbohydrates are essential for energy, and a balanced diet is important for overall health.

Correct: "Regular physical activity can initially help improve your insulin sensitivity and manage your weight."

Regular physical activity is beneficial for improving insulin sensitivity, managing weight, and overall diabetes management.

Incorrect: "You should only take your insulin if your blood sugar levels are above 200 mg/dL."

Insulin should be taken as prescribed by a healthcare provider, not based solely on blood sugar levels at a given moment. Consistent use is important for maintaining stable glucose levels.

Incorrect: "Skipping meals can help you avoid high blood sugar levels."

Skipping meals can lead to unstable blood sugar levels and is not a recommended strategy for managing diabetes. Regular, balanced meals are important.

By using prioritization words like first, most important, and initially, the correct answers emphasize the critical actions needed for effective diabetes management.

Take care of closed-ended Words

When taking the NCLEX-RN, it's important to be cautious of options containing closed-ended words like "all," "always," "every," "must," "none," "never," "only," "absolutely," "certainly," "definite," "totally," "unquestionably," "completely," and "entirely." These words imply an extreme or absolute condition, which is often incorrect in the context of nursing scenarios, where there is usually some variation or flexibility. For example, a question might ask, "What is the correct nursing intervention for a patient experiencing chest pain?" If one of the answers says, "You must always administer oxygen first," it is likely incorrect because "always" implies that there is no other appropriate action under any circumstances, which is rarely the case in nursing.

On the other hand, look for answers with open-ended words like "may," "usually," "normally," "commonly," "generally," "occasionally," "possibly," "sometimes," "frequently," "likely," "often," and "typically." These words suggest that the action may be appropriate in many situations, but not necessarily all. For example, "The nurse should generally assess the patient's vital signs first in cases of chest pain" is more likely to be a correct answer since "generally" acknowledges that the approach may vary depending on the patient's specific situation.

An 82-year-old patient with dementia becomes increasingly agitated in the late afternoon, refusing to take medications and expressing confusion about their surroundings. The nurse needs to decide the most appropriate first intervention.

MCQ:

What should the nurse do first to manage the patient's agitation?

A. "I will administer a sedative immediately to calm the patient."

B. "I will reassure the patient and create a quiet, calming environment."

C. "I will apply restraints to prevent the patient from harming themselves."

D. "I will call the physician to adjust the patient's medication regimen."

Correct Answer:

B. "I will reassure the patient and create a quiet, calming environment."

Explanation:

A. "I will administer a sedative immediately to calm the patient." – This statement uses the word "immediately," implying sedation is the first and necessary action, which is often not the case. Non-pharmacological interventions should be tried first, especially for managing agitation in dementia patients. Sedatives carry risks, and using them too early can mask underlying issues.

B. "I will reassure the patient and create a quiet, calming environment." – This is the correct answer because it focuses on non-invasive, flexible approaches. Dementia patients often respond well to environmental and emotional adjustments. This strategy reflects a gentle, patient-centered approach, which is often the best first step in reducing agitation.

C. "I will apply restraints to prevent the patient from harming themselves." – Restraints are a last resort and should not be the initial intervention. They can increase agitation and distress in dementia patients. This option suggests a rigid and unnecessary escalation of care, making it inappropriate as a first step.

D. "I will call the physician to adjust the patient's medication regimen." – While medication adjustments might be needed later, the nurse should first explore immediate, non-pharmacological solutions to address the current agitation. This option suggests bypassing simpler, more effective strategies in favor of an action that may not be needed right away.

Take care of Prioritization

Situations Requiring Immediate or Urgent Prioritization

These scenarios demand prompt action, as failure to intervene could result in harm or life-threatening conditions for the patient. For instance, if a patient is experiencing a seizure and is expelling mucus while having their tongue roll back, the nurse's first priority should be to clear the airway, ensuring the patient can breathe easily. In such cases, it is not appropriate to simply call the healthcare provider or check vital signs, as those actions could delay critical intervention.

When faced with questions about urgent priorities on the NCLEX, you might encounter options that include contacting a healthcare provider. If there are no immediate nursing interventions that can address the situation effectively or if the scenario is beyond the nurse's capacity to manage, then selecting the option to call the healthcare provider is justified.

Situations Requiring Intermediate Priority

The NCLEX often assesses your clinical judgment and ability to prioritize care. Intermediate priority situations are those that require attention but are not immediately life-threatening. These can often be managed without delaying urgent actions. You can usually identify the urgency of a situation by analyzing the question and the answer choices, which will reveal whether the nurse can manage the task independently.

In this category, you wouldn't select "call the healthcare provider" if there are other actions the nurse can perform to address the issue. For example, checking a patient's vital signs is an intermediate priority that can take place before performing CPR in a situation where the patient has stopped breathing.

Situations Requiring Low Priority

Low-priority situations are those that do not pose an immediate threat to the patient's well-being and can be postponed if higher-priority tasks are necessary. Actions that do not directly contribute to the patient's immediate care fall into this category. For example, repositioning a patient to prevent pressure sores is important but is a lower priority compared to urgent actions like assessing vital signs if the patient is unstable.

When a nurse is managing multiple clients or tasks in an emergency, effective prioritization is essential. This involves evaluating available resources, time constraints, and the severity of each situation to determine the most appropriate order of care. Thus, managing priorities not only relies on clinical judgment but also on understanding the broader context of care delivery in the healthcare setting.

A nurse is caring for a laboring mother who suddenly reports a severe headache and shows signs of elevated blood pressure, indicating potential complications.

MCQ:

What should the nurse do first to manage the situation?

A. "I will administer pain medication to relieve the headache."

B. "I will assess the fetal heart rate to ensure the baby is stable."

C. "I will notify the healthcare provider about the mother's symptoms."

D. "I will check the mother's vital signs and perform a neurological assessment."

Correct Answer:

D. "I will check the mother's vital signs and perform a neurological assessment."

Explanation:

A. "I will administer pain medication to relieve the headache." – This option is incorrect because administering pain medication does not address the potential underlying issue indicated by the severe headache and elevated blood pressure. Before providing medication, the nurse needs to assess the mother's condition to determine the cause of the headache.

B. "I will assess the fetal heart rate to ensure the baby is stable." – While monitoring the fetal heart rate is important, it is not the immediate priority in this situation. The mother's symptoms suggest a potential medical emergency that needs to be addressed first, making this option less appropriate as the initial response.

C. "I will notify the healthcare provider about the mother's symptoms." – Notifying the healthcare provider is essential, but it should occur after conducting an initial assessment. The nurse must first gather vital information about the mother's condition to provide an accurate report to the provider.

D. "I will check the mother's vital signs and perform a neurological assessment." – This is the correct answer because assessing vital signs and conducting a neurological examination are crucial steps to identify any serious complications, such as preeclampsia or other hypertensive disorders. This option prioritizes the immediate safety of the mother and baby, aligning with best nursing practices in this scenario.

Finding options with urgent priority with keywords

You can look for the following words to determine if the action is of urgent priority.

- ✓ Immediate
- ✓ Urgent
- ✓ Active
- ✓ Coma
- ✓ shock
- ✓ uncontrolled
- ✓ bleeding, etc.

When to choose the option ' Call the health care provider'?

If there is any urgent action to be taken which when not immediately intervened can be life-threatening, but can be intervened by the nurse to save that patient, your option must not contain anything that says to call the health care provider. Sometimes, you have to prioritize based on the situation also.

Sometimes, the question may call for a medical emergency that is out of the hands of nursing intervention. In such a situation, you have to choose the option to 'Call for a health care provider'.

Example :

A patient who is kept in observation after a tonsillectomy operation suddenly starts to vomit blood and feels pain in the chest. What should be the first nursing priority?

i. Call the health care provider.
ii. Proning of the patient must be done to increase the SpO2 level.
iii. Give immediately bismuth subsalicylate to stop the vomiting.
iv. Monitor Blood Pressure

We studied to watch out for words like immediately given in option iii. That may lure you to choose the answer. But in this case, it's not because it is a medical emergency condition.

Vomiting blood is considered a medical emergency. You should always contact a medical professional if you notice blood in the vomit. It can be hard to determine the cause and severity of bleeding without a medical opinion. So, your option should be 'Call the health care provider'. If the condition of the patient is critical and needs medical intervention and there is nothing that a nurse can do to save the life of the patient, calling a health care provider would be the best option.

Prioritizing with the focus or strategic words and statements

Often it may seem like all the options of the question presented to you are correct. But you may be asked- 'Which among all those correct options should be given more focus'. This can be understood by the focus words or strategic words.

Examples of these situations:

Que : Situation ……………….What should the nurse do **next**?

Here the focus word is next. If such words are there definitely 'all options are correct' wouldn't be your answer. There is one specific answer which should be followed after the situation described in the question.

Que: Situation ……………….What should the nurse do first?

The situation is given and the examiner is trying to find what will you prioritize at the beginning. In this case, you should eliminate all the options that can be done later or that don't help to save life or ease the current condition of the patient.

Some other statements are:

Which action should be kept on **priority**?
What should be done **immediately**?
Which of the following option is the **best for this situation**?
Which of the actions is **most appropriate**?

A nurse is caring for a patient who was admitted to the emergency department after experiencing a stroke. The patient presents with slurred speech, weakness on the right side, and difficulty swallowing. After a quick assessment, the nurse notes that the patient's blood pressure is elevated, and the healthcare provider has ordered a CT scan to rule out a hemorrhagic stroke. The patient is alert but anxious about the situation.
MCQ Question:
What should the nurse do next?
A. "I will explain the CT scan procedure to the patient to reduce her anxiety."
B. "I will start an IV line to prepare for possible medication administration."
C. "I will assess the patient's neurological status again."
D. "I will notify the healthcare provider about the patient's elevated blood pressure."
Correct Answer:
B. "I will start an IV line to prepare for possible medication administration."
Explanation:
A. "I will explain the CT scan procedure to the patient to reduce her anxiety." – While explaining the procedure is important and can help ease the patient's anxiety, it is not the most immediate priority. The patient's medical condition requires actions that ensure her safety and preparation for further treatment.
B. "I will start an IV line to prepare for possible medication administration." – This is the correct answer. Starting an IV line is a priority because it prepares the patient for any urgent interventions, such as medication administration that may be required after the CT scan results. This action directly addresses the immediate needs of the patient.

C. "I will assess the patient's neurological status again." – Although ongoing assessment of the patient's neurological status is essential in stroke care, this action is not the next step in terms of immediate intervention. The initial assessment has already been performed, and the focus should now be on preparing for treatment.

D. "I will notify the healthcare provider about the patient's elevated blood pressure." – While it is crucial to communicate significant findings to the healthcare provider, this action should be done after ensuring the patient is prepared for further interventions. The elevated blood pressure may require action, but it does not take precedence over preparing for immediate treatment options.

In this scenario, the focus word "next" emphasizes the need for immediate action, allowing the nurse to prioritize starting the IV line to facilitate timely care.

Prioritizing based on any special steps in nursing procedure which you must not escape.

There is some nursing procedure for many conditions that you must not escape or should follow in the same order as prescribed. The examiner is trying to access your knowledge in that particular topic. All the given options could be correct if the order was not there but what the question typically tries to test you is whether you know the particular steps of any nursing process.

This type of prioritization question could be a little hard as it needs your knowledge of the specific topic.

Example :

A patient is showing symptoms of allergic reactions and incompatibility with the blood transfusion. What could be the first nursing intervention?

  i. Change the IV tubing and keep the IV line open to normal saline.
 ii. Stop transfusion immediately.
iii. Obtain urine specimen.
 iv. Notify the blood bank and health care provider.

The correct answer to this question is option number ii.

As soon as a nurse observes a hemolytic reaction, her job is to stop the transfusion immediately and change the IV tubing and keep the IV line open to the normal saline. She then notifies the blood bank and the health care provider about the reaction and monitors and records the vital signs of the patient. If there is any emergency medicine that is given and obtains urine specimen is. All the tubings, labels, blood bags, etc should be returned to the blood bank after documenting everything.

Prioritizing based on ABC

One of the easiest priority-based situations is seeing the ABC. Patients with problems with the airway, breathing, and circulation should always be the priority, and it should always be in that order.

The priority should be seeing if there is any obstruction in the airway, next is seeing if there is breathing, then circulation. That means, if you are given multiple options of checking blood pressure, or lungs auscultation or checking airways, your priority should be checking the airways.

Example :

The patient with a diagnosis of esophageal cancer is receiving morphine sulfate subcutaneously for the management of pain. When preparing the plan of care for the client, the nurse includes which priority action?

   i. Monitor any blood in the sputum.
   ii. Monitor blood pressure.
   iii. Treat with naloxone as an antidote to morphine for treating the side effect.
   iv. Ask the patient to cough and take deep breaths.

Respiratory depression is potentially the most serious side effect induced by morphine sulfate. So, what can be done to ensure there is adequate care?

You should watch out for clearance of the airways and see if the patient is breathing properly. To ensure this, the last option says to the patient to cough and take deep breathing should be done should be your answer.

Monitoring BP is the only third option in ABC. And the priority action is still to ensure the breathing is correct. Option 1 is not suitable for the situation of the question. Option 3 is also wrong although the antidote of morphine sulfate is naloxone, nothing is mentioned that there is any side effect to the patient. In any situation prioritizing based on ABC that is caring and giving priority to airways, breathing, and circulation should be done.

Prioritizing based on CABC

Prioritizing based on ABC procedure doesn't always necessarily be true. If there is a need for cardiopulmonary resuscitation or CPR, the correct order would be CABC in which the first C stands for CPR. Cardiopulmonary Resuscitation is an emergency lifesaving procedure performed when the heart stops beating.

Example :

Consider a situation in which the ECG shows the readings of myocardial infraction, the person is unconscious and stops breathing. Which of the priority action must be done first?

    i.   clearing out the airways,
    ii.   giving CPR,
    iii.   checking vital signs,
    iv.   calling health care provider immediately etc,

Ans: giving CPR because this action is of high priority.

Prioritizing based on Maslow's hierarchy of needs.

Another technique to prioritize is using Maslow's hierarchy of needs. Maslow mentioned that there are 5 levels of needs of the individuals which can be translated for our use in prioritizing the needs of the patients.

1. Physiological needs
2. Safety needs
3. Social needs
4. Esteem
5. Self-Actualization

Physiological needs are those needs that are needed for survival. You should omit all other answers if there is an option in priority that mentions the survival needs.

Examples of physiological needs are:
- Nutrition
- Oxygen
- Clothes
- Shelter

Safety Needs are associated with privacy, health, and property.

Social Needs- family and friends come here.

Esteem covers respect, giving confidence to the patients, making them feel good, etc.

Self- Actualization- Things like morality, humanity, creativity, etc falls into this domain.

Example :

After a successful operation on the lung tumor, the client is feeling restless and is complaining that he is feeling a little difficulty in breathing, what could be your nursing intervention?

   i. Tell him that such symptom is normal after the operation and pacify him.
   ii. Tell the caretakers about the client's situation and that they are trying their best to ease the situation.
   iii. Do not share any details about the patient's condition with the family.
   iv. Check ABG and keep the patient on oxygen

The answer to this situation is quite simple. There is a priority here. The client is already feeling difficulty breathing. If there would be any option like calling for the assistance of a health care provider, that could be a better option but here, the last option talks about physiological needs. The second and third options are incorrect as they talk about safety needs. The first is an incorrect answer, remember the main mantra of prioritization, you should prioritize based on the client's need and the client's situation, not what you think. Also, this point is trying to make the patient feel safe and better. There are better options.

Example : A nurse observes that the patient is suffering from anorexia due to the side effect of drug X and has lost a lot of weight in 2 months. Which of the following options will be best for her to look out for first for caring for the patient?

    i.   Discuss with the health care provider to reduce the dose of the drug.
    ii.   Tell the patient to stop taking the drug unless prescribed by the health care worker again.
    iii. Watch out for caring for malnutrition.
    iv. Instruct him that side effect is normal and not to worry about any physical appearance.

Correct Ans- Option iii.

Option 2 is wrong ethically you cannot tell the patient to stop the drug unless prescribed by the physician.
Option 1 is wrong though seems a good and collaborative approach.
option 4 seems a better answer. But in the priority, you have to treat malnutrition as the patient has quickly lost a lot of weight.

Example :

A nurse is assigned to 4 different clients (hypothetical). Which of these clients needs the least priority based on the situational description?

    i.   A patient suspected of MI has stopped breathing.
    ii.   A lung tuberculosis patient who wants support with her bed elevation.
    iii. A patient who is feeling dizzy after falling due to low BP.
    iv. A patient is admitted with a history of seizures with secretions coming out of the mouth.

The correct answer to this question is answer number 2. It's quite clear that she is not in any life-threatening situation and also this condition is not directly linked to the disease she is in.

Other all options are either of high or intermediate priority.

Ok. let me change the question.

Can you prioritize the nursing actions?

Ok, So from the least prioritization, we already know that option number 2 is of low priority.

So, what could be number one? We have to follow CABC which is a slight modification of ABC. C before ABC stands for CPR and this is done to patients who have stopped breathing if it continues for some minutes, the patient may die so the number 1 priority should be option no 1. The patient has stopped breathing so needs immediate CPR.

So, which option is the next?

Remember CABC. The second option is Clearing the Airways. The question mentions that there is mucus secretion with seizure. Such patients may also have their tongue rolled up blocking the airway. We have to pull the tongue out or clear out the secretions. This could be of second-priority case.

Next is option 3. The patient is feeling dizzy and has a low BP. This is a circulatory issue. So, given an option to choose the patient case in an emergency between these 4 patients, the order mentioned should be followed.

Prioritization with Emergency Department Triage

Think of a situation in which you are in the emergency department and you are assigned to different clients. There is a shortage of manpower and there is a rush of patients due to some big bus accident. How would you prioritize the situation? Would you save women first or babies first? Would you prioritize old people first? What are the criteria for prioritizatio?

We can classify the cases into 3 groups:

i. Highest Priority Clients.
ii. Urgent Priority Clients and
iii. Non Urgent Clients

Emergent or Highest Priority Clients (Red Zone)

If the clients have chances of survival with nursing intervention and need some immediate attention and if it is a life and death issue of care, such patients need the highest caring priority.

So, who could be the patient falling in the highest priority of care?

- ✓ Patients with acute heart conditions such as Myocardial infarction.
- ✓ Stroke,
- ✓ Clients with amputated limbs
- ✓ Acute chemical effect on eyes
- ✓ Acute respiratory attacks such as Asthma, or any anaphylactic reaction.
- ✓ Patients complaining of chest pain, burns, hypersensitive reactions, etc

Urgent or Intermediate Priority (Yellow Zone)

In this case, those clients who have non-life threatening injuries are put. One rule is they have to get medical service within 30 minutes to 120 minutes.

An example of such a case is a patient with

- ✓ Open fracture,
- ✓ Wounds
- ✓ Medium burns

Non-urgent or Least Priority (Green Zone)

In this zone, those patients who do not have life-threatening complications and who have local injuries and can wait for 2 hours for a healthcare worker are put in.

Examples of clients with such cases are :

- ✓ Muscle Strain
- ✓ Ligament Strain
- ✓ Closed fracture, etc.

Example :

An emergency department nurse has to prioritize among different clients rushing into an emergency department due to a bus accident. Which of the following cases should you prioritize first if there is a serious lack of nurses in the facility?

   i. Client with amputated left leg.
   ii. Client with an open fracture of right ulnar bone.
   iii. Client with laceration of the palm.
   iv. Client with close fracture of the tibia.

The question is about priority so there must be only one answer. According to the emergency department triage, patients who have life-threatening situations and need immediate attention are placed in Emergent Priority or Highest Priority care. So the correct answer for this question is Option number i or client with an amputated leg.

If he or she is not treated, the patient may go under heavy blood loss and shock.

Similarly, patients with open fracture come under second priority or Urgent Priority and Patient with laceration of the palm and close fracture falls in 3rd or non-urgent priority.

Eliminating similar options

In many cases, you will be given many options which sound alike or convey the same meaning or situations. There will however be one option that would be quite different from the rest. If you cannot figure out the correct option, try out your luck, the option with a different answer will be your answer. All you have to do is eliminate all the similar options that convey quite the same meaning.

Case: Mr. Johnstone, a 72-year-old patient, visits the ambulatory care clinic for follow-up after experiencing mild weakness and difficulty walking. He has a history of hypertension and mild osteoarthritis. The nurse assesses him and provides guidance on maintaining mobility and improving safety during ambulation. The nurse also educates Mr. Johnstone about managing his chronic conditions and preventing complications related to decreased mobility.

Multiple Choice Question:
Question: Which of the following statements made by the nurse are correct regarding the care of ambulatory patients? (Select two options)
Options:
"Avoid physical activity entirely to prevent falls and joint damage."
"Using a walker or cane can improve your balance and reduce the risk of falls."
"It is important to remain active, but take frequent breaks to avoid overexertion."
"Only engage in physical activity when you are completely pain-free."

"Physical activity should focus on strengthening muscles and improving flexibility."
"Limit activity to a minimum, as any movement could worsen your condition."
Answer Explanation:
"Avoid physical activity entirely to prevent falls and joint damage."
Wrong. This option suggests complete inactivity, which is not recommended. For ambulatory patients, maintaining some level of physical activity is crucial to prevent muscle atrophy, joint stiffness, and worsening of mobility. Avoiding all activity can actually lead to increased risk of falls and further complications.
"Using a walker or cane can improve your balance and reduce the risk of falls."
Correct. This is a recommended strategy in many cases, especially for patients with mobility or balance issues. Assistive devices like walkers and canes help stabilize patients during ambulation, reducing the risk of falls and improving independence.
"It is important to remain active, but take frequent breaks to avoid overexertion."
Correct. This advice is sound for ambulatory patients. Staying active is important to maintain physical strength and mobility, but frequent breaks are essential to prevent overexertion, especially in elderly patients or those with chronic conditions.
"Only engage in physical activity when you are completely pain-free."
Wrong. Expecting to be completely pain-free before engaging in physical activity is unrealistic for many patients with chronic conditions such as arthritis. Pain management strategies should be in place, but complete avoidance of activity can worsen mobility issues.
"Physical activity should focus on strengthening muscles and improving flexibility."
Wrong. While this statement is partially correct, it's not one of the best choices for this question. Strengthening muscles and improving flexibility are important, but the primary focus for ambulatory patients should be on maintaining safe mobility and balance. The emphasis should also include avoiding overexertion.
"Limit activity to a minimum, as any movement could worsen your condition."
Wrong. Similar to option 1, this advice contradicts the principles of promoting mobility and preventing complications such as muscle weakness and joint stiffness. Reduced movement can lead to a rapid decline in a patient's overall physical condition.
Strategy: Eliminating Similar Options
In this question, several options promote extreme limitations on physical activity (Options 1, 4, and 6), which can be grouped as similar statements that contradict common nursing advice for ambulatory patients. Since they all suggest avoiding or severely limiting physical activity, they can be eliminated, leaving Options 2, 3, and 5. Among these, Options 2 and 3 stand out as more directly related to safe ambulation and overall mobility, making them the correct answers.

TYPES OF QUESTION FORMAT IN NEXT GENERATION NCLEX

The questions in the new next generation NCLEX are similar to old format but with addition of case study questions and additional stand alone questions.

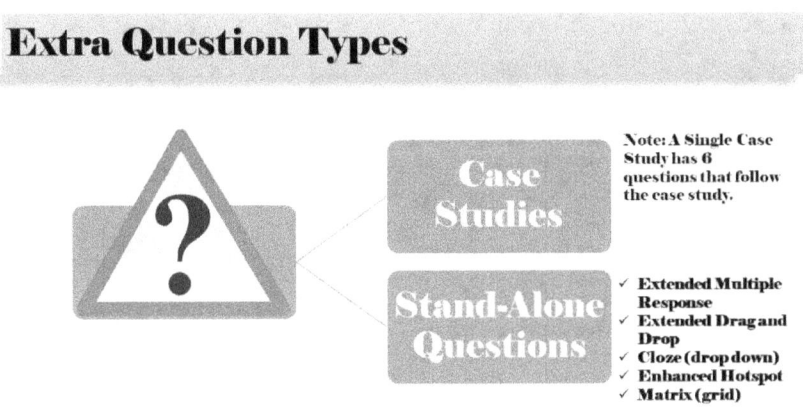

Case Studies in NGN

In the Next Generation NCLEX (NGN), case studies are crafted to mimic real-world patient care scenarios. Each scenario typically features a patient dealing with certain symptoms or a medical condition. You'll be asked various questions that challenge you to use clinical reasoning and make informed decisions. The main objective is to test how well you can identify important signs, evaluate the information, rank potential diagnoses, come up with appropriate interventions, and assess the results.

Stand-Alone Questions

Stand-alone questions are separate from case studies and come as individual questions. While they also evaluate clinical judgment, these questions use a more standard approach. Formats can include multiple-choice, select-all-that-apply, or other question types. These questions focus on specific aspects of clinical decision-making and require you to draw from your medical knowledge to answer correctly.

Case Study Question : Introduction

The Next Generation NCLEX (NGN) maintains some aspects of the previous exam format but introduces new elements, including case study and standalone questions. These changes are intended to assess candidates' clinical judgment and decision-making abilities in a more comprehensive and practical way.

A key feature of the NGN is the use of case study questions, which are designed to test a candidate's ability to apply critical thinking in realistic patient situations. Each case study consists of six questions related to a specific scenario, which includes the patient's health history, nurse's notes, vital signs, lab results, and medications.

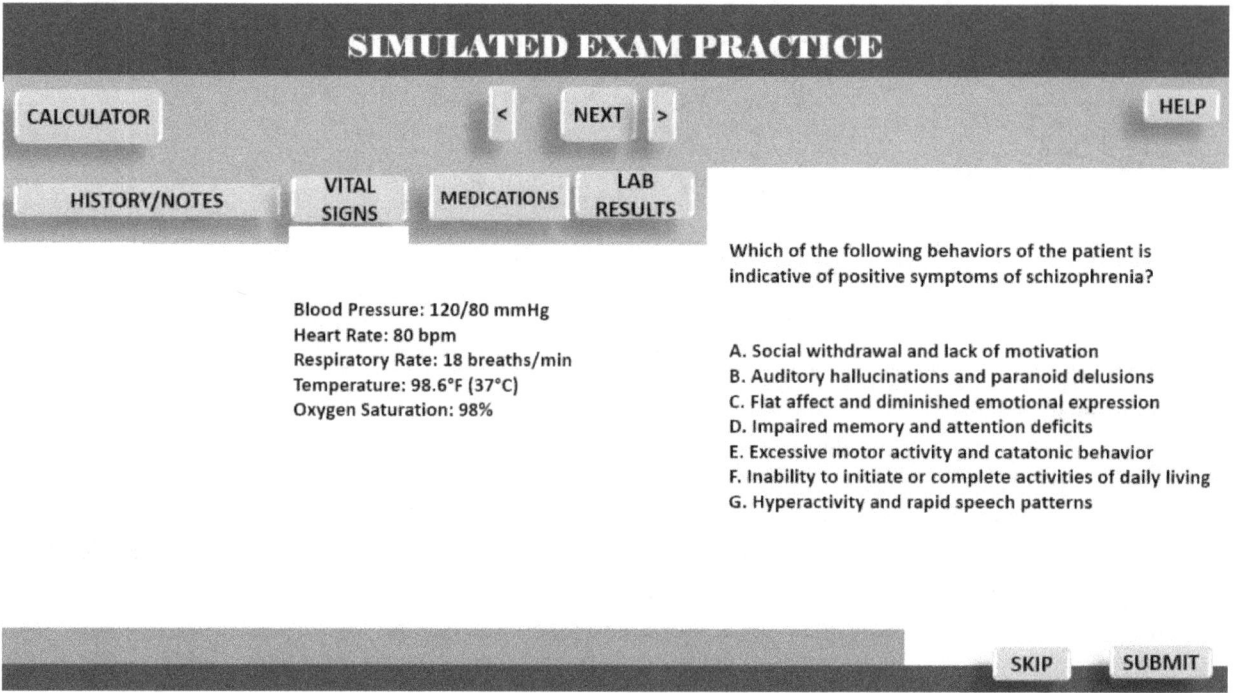

During the exam, case study questions are presented on the right side of the screen with multiple choice answers. As candidates respond to each question, the next question in the series appears on the right side, continuing with the same case study. These six questions evaluate a range of cognitive skills, including:

- Identifying relevant cues
- Analyzing these cues
- Prioritizing potential hypotheses
- Developing solutions
- Implementing appropriate actions
- Assessing outcomes

What do these cognitive skills entail?

Recognition of Cues: This skill involves identifying important information or indicators from a given scenario or case study. Example: In a patient case study, noticing signs such as an elevated heart rate, difficulty breathing, and chest pain as potential indicators of a cardiovascular problem.

Analysis of Cues: This refers to the ability to examine and interpret the identified cues to understand their relevance and implications. Example: After identifying the signs mentioned above, analyzing them to determine that they might suggest a possible heart attack or myocardial infarction.

Prioritization of Hypotheses: This skill involves ranking or ordering potential explanations or hypotheses based on the analyzed cues. Example: Evaluating different possible causes for the patient's symptoms and prioritizing the likelihood of a heart attack over other possibilities like anxiety or digestive issues.

Generation of Solutions: This entails devising and proposing possible actions or solutions based on the prioritized hypotheses. Example: If a heart attack is deemed the most likely explanation, potential solutions might include administering aspirin, calling for emergency medical help, and preparing for possible cardiac procedures.

Taking Appropriate Action: This involves executing the chosen intervention or solution based on the prioritized hypotheses. Example: Implementing the necessary steps such as contacting emergency services, giving aspirin, and arranging for the patient's transport to a medical facility for further assessment and treatment.

Evaluation of Outcomes: This skill involves reviewing the results or effectiveness of the actions taken and determining any further steps required. Example: After the patient has received medical care, evaluating the results means checking if the interventions improved the patient's condition, monitoring for any side effects, and modifying the care plan if needed.

To excel in the NGN exam, candidates should adopt a structured approach for tackling case study questions. This method involves thoroughly reviewing the case study details, identifying key cues, analyzing these cues to form prioritized hypotheses, developing solutions based on these hypotheses, implementing appropriate actions, and assessing the outcomes.

For example, if a case study involves a patient with severe abdominal pain, the candidate should first identify relevant cues such as vital signs, medical history, and medications. By analyzing these cues, potential diagnoses like appendicitis or gastroenteritis can be considered. Following this, the candidate would formulate a plan, monitor its effectiveness through the patient's response, and adjust the approach as necessary.

Effective Strategies for Handling Case Studies

1. Thorough Reading: Start by carefully reading the entire case study to build a strong foundation. This includes understanding the patient's medical history, symptoms, and vital signs. Example: For a case study involving chest pain, ensure you grasp details such as the pain's duration, characteristics, associated symptoms, and any relevant past medical conditions like heart disease or diabetes.

2. Problem Identification: Identify the primary issue or medical condition impacting the patient. This step is crucial for prioritizing interventions and addressing the most critical aspects effectively. Example: In a case where the patient experiences shortness of breath, determine if the issue is respiratory, cardiac, or due to other factors to guide appropriate interventions.

3. Application of Nursing Knowledge: Utilize your nursing knowledge to connect symptoms with potential causes and underlying factors. This involves applying your understanding of anatomy, physiology, and pathophysiology. Example: In a case study involving altered mental status, use your nursing expertise to explore possible causes such as hypoxia, metabolic disturbances, or neurological issues.

4. Multiple Perspectives: Examine the case study from various viewpoints, including the patient's perspective, the healthcare team's perspective, and any ethical or legal considerations. This helps to broaden your understanding and enhances critical thinking. Example: If a patient refuses a prescribed treatment, consider the situation from the patient's autonomy, the healthcare team's duty to provide the best care, and any legal or ethical implications regarding informed consent.

5. Plan of Care Development: Create a comprehensive care plan based on the identified problem and associated issues. Focus on evidence-based interventions that address the patient's needs and fit the healthcare context. Example: For a patient with diabetes and a foot ulcer, develop a plan that includes wound care, glycemic control, patient education, and coordination with other healthcare professionals.

Extended Multiple options or Multiple Answer Questions

Multiple options or multiple answers for a single type of question.

Extended means there would be many options.

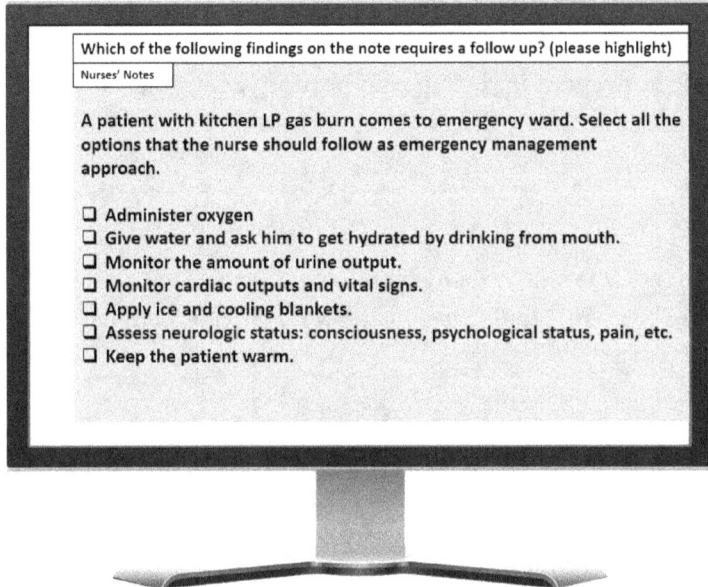

Note:

- For multiple-response questions, there is a partial marking system.
- You get marks for all the right options selected, unlike the previous system where candidates get 0 marks even when a single option is incorrect.

Strategies for extended multiple answers questions:

The Multiple Answer Case Study questions in the Next Gen NCLEX exam require you to identify all the correct answers to a particular scenario or problem. To effectively solve such questions, you can follow these step-by-step approaches:

1. **Understand the scenario and question:**

Read the case study scenario carefully, identify the key issues, and determine the type of question being asked. It is important to understand the context and what is being asked of you to choose the correct answers.

Example:

A case study scenario might describe a patient with heart failure who is prescribed multiple medications, and the question might ask which medications should be withheld if the patient has a low blood pressure reading.

2. **Identify possible answers:**

After understanding the scenario and question, generate a list of possible answers by reviewing your knowledge and the given information. It is essential to review all options before selecting the correct answers.

Example:

In the heart failure case study scenario, possible answers might include all the medications the patient is taking, as well as additional medications that could potentially affect blood pressure.

3. **Eliminate incorrect answers:**

Review each option and eliminate those that are not relevant or do not apply to the scenario. Consider the context of the scenario and the question being asked. This step helps to narrow down your options and select the correct answers.

Example:

In the heart failure case study scenario, medications that do not affect blood pressure or have no direct effect on heart failure management could be eliminated as incorrect answers.

4. **Select the correct answers:**

After eliminating incorrect answers, identify the correct answers by choosing the options that directly apply to the scenario and the question being asked. Review your choices and ensure that you have selected all the correct options.

Example:

In the heart failure case study scenario, the correct answers might include medications that lower blood pressure, such as diuretics and ACE inhibitors, and should be withheld if the patient's blood pressure is low.

5. **Check for accuracy:**

Before submitting your answers, review your choices to ensure that they are accurate and complete. Check if you have selected all the correct options.

Example:

In the heart failure case study scenario, double-check to ensure that all medications that lower blood pressure have been selected, and none that do not affect blood pressure have been chosen.
Let's solve another extended multiple answers question.

QUE: A patient with heart failure is taking multiple medications. Which of the following medications should be withheld if the patient has a low blood pressure reading? Select all that apply.

A) Furosemide

B) Digoxin

C) Lisinopril

D) Spironolactone

E) Metoprolol

Correct Answers:

A) Furosemide C) Lisinopril

Explanation:

A. Furosemide is a diuretic medication that helps reduce fluid buildup in the body and lower blood pressure. If a patient with heart failure has a low blood pressure reading, withholding furosemide would help avoid a further reduction in blood pressure.

B) Digoxin is a medication that strengthens the heart's contractions and is used to treat heart failure. However, it does not directly affect blood pressure and does not need to be withheld if a patient has a low blood pressure reading.

C) Lisinopril is an ACE inhibitor medication that lowers blood pressure and is commonly used to treat heart failure. If a patient has a low blood pressure reading, withholding lisinopril would help avoid a further reduction in blood pressure.

D) Spironolactone is a potassium-sparing diuretic that helps reduce fluid buildup in the body and lower blood pressure. However, it is not as potent as furosemide in reducing blood pressure, and its use should be evaluated based on the patient's overall condition and clinical presentation.

E) Metoprolol is a beta-blocker medication that lowers blood pressure and is used to treat heart failure. However, it is not as potent as furosemide or lisinopril in reducing blood pressure, and its use should be evaluated based on the patient's overall condition and clinical presentation.

In summary, Furosemide and Lisinopril are the correct answers to this question as they are both medications that can significantly reduce blood pressure and should be withheld if the patient has a low blood pressure reading. The other options may also be used to treat heart failure, but do not need to be withheld specifically for low blood pressure.

Extended Drag and Drop Questions

- Instead of clicking all the right options which could be multiple right options, you have to drag and drop the right options in the space provided.

- May be useful in questions that ask you to arrange tasks by priority.

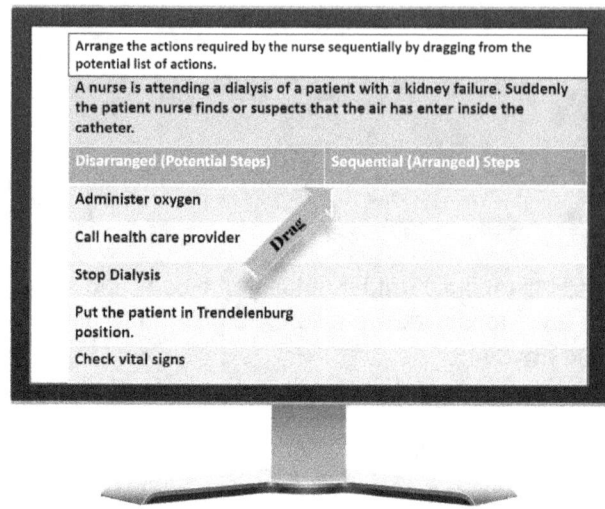

Strategy for solving 'Extended drag-and-drop questions:

Extended drag-and-drop type questions are becoming increasingly popular on the Next Generation NCLEX RN exam. These questions require test takers to not only select the correct answer but also to place the answers in the correct order or context. Below are some strategies to effectively approach extended drag-and-drop questions, along with a case study and example of nursing care for a patient who has drowned.

Read the question and instructions carefully: Make sure to read the question stem and any accompanying instructions carefully. These questions can be complex and it is important to understand what is being asked before attempting to answer.

Identify the key concepts: Identify the key concepts or pieces of information that the question is testing. For example, in the case study below, the key concepts might include drowning, nursing care, and patient assessment.

Review all answer options: Read through all answer options carefully, and try to eliminate any that are incorrect. Then, read through the remaining options and consider their relevance to the key concepts identified in step 2.

Determine the correct order: If the question requires the answers to be placed in a specific order, take time to determine the correct order. Often, the order will be provided in the question stem or the instructions.

Practice: Practice is key for mastering extended drag-and-drop questions. Practice answering questions in this format to become comfortable with the process and identify any areas of weakness.

Now, let's look at an example of a case study for nursing care for a patient who has drowned:

Case Study: Nursing Care for Drowning Patient

Mr. Smith, a 54-year-old man, is brought to the emergency department after being pulled from a swimming pool. He is unresponsive and has no pulse. The healthcare team performs cardiopulmonary resuscitation (CPR) and is able to restore a pulse. Mr. Smith is admitted to the hospital and transferred to the medical-surgical unit for ongoing care.

Drag and drop the following nursing interventions in the correct order for Mr. Smith's care:

- Assess Mr. Smith's airway and breathing
- Monitor Mr. Smith's vital signs
- Administer oxygen as needed
- Obtain a chest x-ray to evaluate lung function
- Provide emotional support to Mr. Smith and his family

Answer:

1. Assess Mr. Smith's airway and breathing
2. Administer oxygen as needed
3. Obtain a chest x-ray to evaluate lung function
4. Monitor Mr. Smith's vital signs
5. Provide emotional support to Mr. Smith and his family

Explanation:

In this case, the key concepts are nursing care for a patient who has drowned, and the order of nursing interventions for Mr. Smith's care. The correct order is to first assess Mr. Smith's airway and breathing, then administer oxygen as needed, obtain a chest x-ray to evaluate lung function, monitor vital signs, and finally provide emotional support to Mr. Smith and his family. This order ensures that the most urgent needs are addressed first, followed by ongoing monitoring and emotional support.

Cloze Type Questions

You will be given a report where there are dropdown options among which you have to choose any phrase that may require immediate intervention or is asking for any actions.

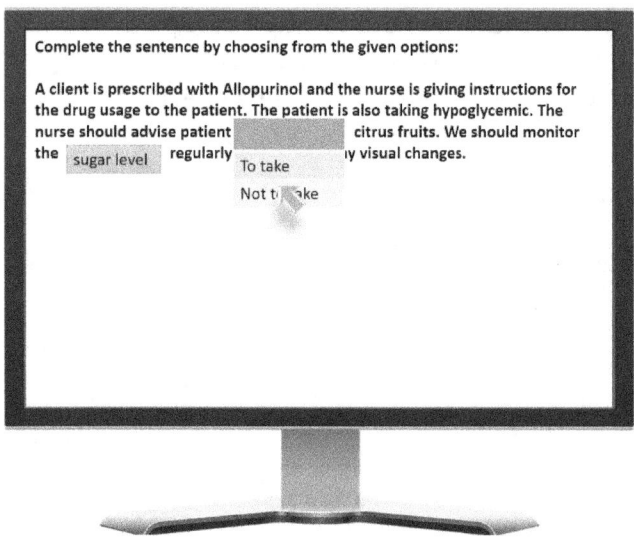

Cloze-type questions require test-takers to fill in the missing words or phrases within a given sentence or passage. To approach such questions effectively, you should consider the context, use your prior knowledge, and eliminate any answer choices that don't fit.

Let's take an example of a nursing care scenario for the lymphatic system to demonstrate how to solve a cloze-type question in the next-generation NCLEX RN exam.

Case Study: Nursing Care for the Lymphatic System

A patient was admitted to the hospital with lymphedema. The nurse caring for the patient should assess the affected limb's size, _____, and skin integrity. The nurse should avoid using tight clothing or _____ on the affected limb, as it can exacerbate the swelling. The nurse should also teach the patient to perform _____ exercises to promote lymphatic drainage.
To solve this cloze-type question, follow these steps:

Read the entire passage or sentence to understand the context and the purpose of the question. In this case, the passage describes nursing care for a patient with lymphedema.

Look for the missing words and phrases, and try to fill them in using your prior knowledge and the context of the passage. For example, in the first sentence, the nurse should assess the affected limb's size, _____, and skin integrity. Based on your prior knowledge of nursing care, you can infer that the missing word is "texture," as it is crucial to assess the texture of the affected limb's skin.

Eliminate answer choices that do not fit. In the second sentence, the nurse should avoid using tight clothing or _____ on the affected limb, as it can exacerbate the swelling. You can eliminate the answer choices that do not make sense in the context of the passage, such as "loose clothing" or "warm compresses." The correct answer is "jewelry," as it can be tight-fitting and put pressure on the affected limb.

Use your prior knowledge and the context of the passage to fill in the remaining missing words or phrases. For example, in the third sentence, the nurse should also teach the patient to perform _____ exercises to promote lymphatic drainage. You can infer that the missing word is "range-of-motion," as exercises that involve moving the affected limb can help promote lymphatic drainage.

So, to solve cloze-type questions in the next-generation NCLEX RN exam, it's essential to read the passage or sentence carefully, use your prior knowledge and the context of the question, and eliminate answer choices that do not fit. By following these steps, you can approach cloze-type questions effectively and increase your chances of getting the correct answer.

Matrix/ Grid Type Questions

A matrix or grid question is a type of question that presents a table or a grid with rows and columns. Each row and column contains a different element that must be matched or evaluated.

This type of question is commonly used in nursing exams, including the NCLEX RN exam. To effectively answer a matrix question, it's important to read the instructions carefully and understand what is being asked. You should also pay close attention to the headings of each row and column, as they provide important information about what you are evaluating.

In the given figure, the column contains any information on the patient's conditions or actions of nurses. The other 3 columns will contain the options for correct and incorrect answers. We will have to select one of the columns.

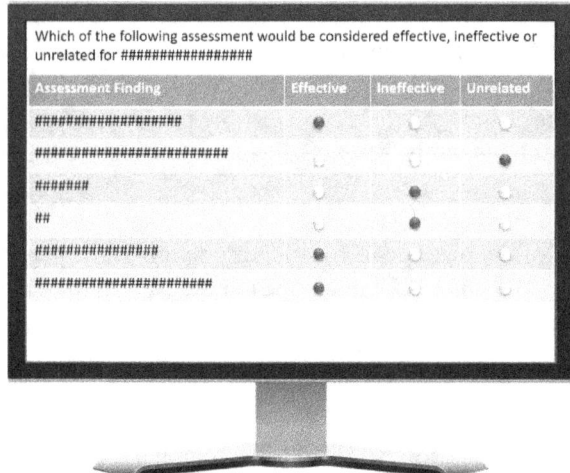

Case study: Ms. Jones is a 65-year-old patient who was admitted to the hospital with complaints of abdominal pain, nausea, and vomiting. She has a history of peptic ulcer disease and takes proton pump inhibitors to manage her symptoms. The physician has ordered a clear liquid diet for Ms. Jones until her symptoms improve.

Instructions: Evaluate the nursing interventions listed below and place them in the appropriate category based on their effectiveness for managing Ms. Jones' digestive symptoms.

Nursing Intervention	Effective	Ineffective	Unrelated
Administering antiemetic medication			
Encouraging Ms. Jones to ambulate in the hallway			

Providing clear liquid diet as ordered			
Administering antacid medication			
Instructing Ms. Jones to avoid caffeine and alcohol			
Applying a heating pad to Ms. Jones' abdomen			

In this example, the nursing interventions are listed in the first column, and the headings for each category (effective, ineffective, and unrelated) are listed in the top row. To answer the question, you would need to evaluate each nursing intervention and determine whether it is effective, ineffective, or unrelated for managing Ms. Jones' digestive symptoms.
Here are some possible answers for each nursing intervention:

- Administering antiemetic medication: Effective

- Encouraging Ms. Jones to ambulate in the hallway: Unrelated

- Providing clear liquid diet as ordered: Effective

- Administering antacid medication: Effective

- Instructing Ms. Jones to avoid caffeine and alcohol: Effective

- Applying a heating pad to Ms. Jones' abdomen: Ineffective

As you can see, the effective interventions are those that are likely to improve Ms. Jones' digestive symptoms, while the ineffective interventions are those that are unlikely to improve her symptoms or may even make them worse. The unrelated interventions are those that do not have a direct impact on Ms. Jones' digestive symptoms.

To prepare for matrix questions on the NCLEX RN exam, it's important to review nursing interventions for different patient scenarios and practice categorizing them based on their effectiveness. You can also review sample NCLEX RN exam questions to get a better idea of how matrix questions are structured and what types of nursing interventions may be included in them.

Highlighting

The answer has to be selected by highlighting the text or sentences.

- You may see a part of medical report (which could be medical or patient history)
- You have to select the words and phrases inside that resemble the need of the question.

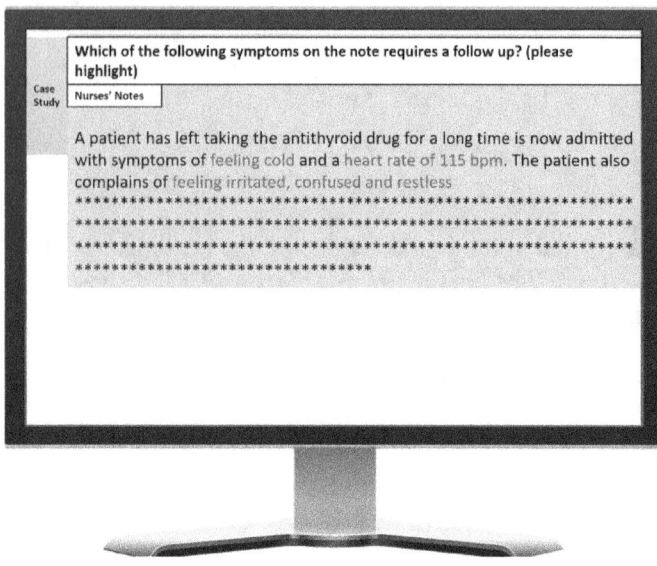

Other Conventional Types of Questions that are the same as the old model are:

- Multiple Choice Questions
- Figure Questions
- Chart/ Table Type Questions
- Audio/Video Questions
- Fill in the blanks type Questions
- Multiple Response Questions

Other Question Types for Standalone Questions

Multiple Choice Question

Most of the question that you will face in the NCLEX examination falls in this category. Many tricks can be applied while answering the multiple-choice question. Many of these tips will be is dealt on a lecture on priority-based questions.

Some tips for your understanding-

   i. Never choose – Call the health care provider as an option if the situation can be managed by a nurse and should be handled quickly to save the life of the patient.
   ii. Never choose all of the above or none of the above as an option if there are keywords like Next, First, or any procedure-related question.
   iii. Look for specific nursing procedures. for example, look for ABG or First look for airways, then breathing, and then circulation if this is an ABG-related question asking you for the next procedure to be followed.
   iv. Look for Maslow's hierarchy of needs while answering a question that asks you to follow when there is any specific need of the patient. For example, if there is any physiological need, that should be followed first before any safety needs or esteem or making the patient feel good. There is a hierarchy of processes while following Maslow's law and this should be followed properly.

We look at all these cases with examples in the lectures of prioritizing answers. This was just for the revision of basic tips that can be taken while selecting the answers for multiple-choice questions.

Figure Questions

In these types of questions, you are given a figure which could be a graph or picture.

Generally, I would suggest you give proper emphasis to the EKG interpretation chapter as a lot of probable questions of this type may come based on what you learn there.

Sometimes, you may also be asked to point out or select the definite part of the figure to choose the correct answer.

Example:

A patient is showing a symptom of an extremely high heart rate of around 250 BPM, low BP, shortness of breath, etc. Upon monitoring via cardiac telemetry, the EKG reading shows the 'saw tooth' appearance with multiple P waves for each QRS complex. Can you identify the cardiac condition of this patient?

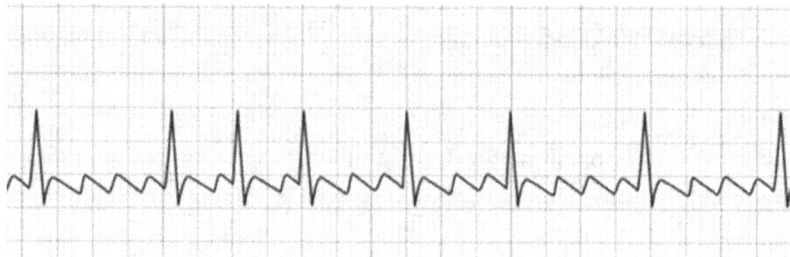

    i.   The EKG shows Atrial Flutter
    ii.   The EKG shows Atrial Fibrillation
    iii. This is a Normal sinus
    iv. EKG shows Sinus Bradycardia

Let's first start with the elimination strategy.

Let's see the options. We are given here that the heart rate is very high at around 250 BPM, so the term bradycardia which means low heartbeat of fewer than 60 beats per minute should be eliminated.

We are left with 3 options, 1, 2, and 3. Again, as an elimination strategy, it's too easy to point out that this is not a normal sinus rhythm. The normal sinus rhythm contains normal P wave, QRS complex, and T wave. Normal sinus is the rhythm of a normal person. Is the patient's condition normal here?

No, the symptoms and the nature of ekg strip are not normal so we have to eliminate this one.

We are now left with options 1 and 2.

This question needs specialized knowledge.

If you are new to interpreting the EKG waves. Don't worry. We will practice that with lots of case studies and examples in the relevant section. Just for your knowledge,

In atrial flutter, there is a coordinated electrical activity in the heart. The rate is regular which means the waves look regular but the p wave shows a saw tooth pattern like the one shown in this graph.

So, the correct answer to this question is option 1 or atrial flutter.

Next for option 2, in atrial fibrillation, there is no coordinated electrical activity. The P waves are absent and blunt waves are seen.

The ecg wave or ekg wave looks something like this. Note in this figure that unlike in atrial flutter, there is no regular rhythm and p waves are absent. There are wavy structures that we cannot distinguish from any kind of wave.

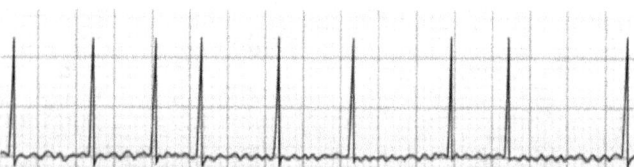

Chart/Table Type Questions

Here, you will be given a chart with some description that may contain the right or the wrong options. You will be prompted to choose the right or wrong options based on the situation.

Example:

A nurse notes down the following symptoms of the patient.

1. the patient has severe hypotension

2. there is a progressive stupor or coma

3. Has electrolyte imbalance upon investigation (decreased sodium level, increased potassium, decreased cortisol, etc)

4. There is dehydration and hypovolemia

Which of these pairs (column) could be correct for the diagnosis and management of this condition?

Diagnosis	Primary Management
Addisonian crisis	IV hydrocortisone
Addison's disease	Hormone Replacement
Cushing syndrome	Potassium Sparing diuretics (Spironolactone)
Cushing syndrome	Hormone Replacement

So, in this question, you have these 4 pairs for the type of disease diagnosis and primary management. The correct answer for this is option no, 1. This is the Addisonian crisis.

Just for your quick knowledge,

Addison's disease is a condition in which there is hypo secretion of adrenocortical hormone and in which the patient shows the following condition. You can memorize this as a 3s condition.

The blood profile shows salt or electrolyte imbalance, there is Sugar or metabolic imbalance and there is sexual imbalance.

Cushing syndrome is hypersecretion of adrenocortical hormone and basically, the symptoms of diabetes are common in cushing syndrome. As a memory tip, understand that there is a 3P-

i. **Polydipsia** or increase in hunger,

ii. **Polyuria** or increase in urination,
iii. **Polyphagia** or increase in appetite etc.

Addisonian crisis is a life-threatening emergency of Addison's disease which comes with all the conditions mentioned in the question like

- ✓ severe hypotension
- ✓ progressive stupor or coma
- ✓ electrolyte imbalance upon investigation (decreased sodium level, increased potassium, decreased cortisol, etc.)
- ✓ dehydration and hypovolemia, etc.

The primary management of this condition is IV hydrocortisone. If you are asked how to administer hydrocortisone, two third the dose should be given in AM and one-third of the dose is given in PM to mimic the normal diurnal rhythm of the body.

We then taper the dose and withdraw.

So, your option for this question is quite clear. You have to select the first option.

Fill in the blanks type question

While it is not as popular as multiple choice and other types of questions you can still expect some fill-in-the-blanks type of questions in your NCLEX examination.

The calculation-based question is used for filling in the purpose of the blank as you need to input the correct answer to some mathematical dosage calculations or other types of questions. You may also be asked to round up the number to some decimal places if the calculation-based question is asked.

See these tips to round up:

- ✓ rounded up to one decimal place: A.B
- ✓ rounded up to two decimal places: A.BC

If the number behind the decimal is more than 5, it is rounded up to the next whole number

for example, if the calculation is 3.87 and you are asked to round up to one decimal place, your choice should be 3.9, not 3.8.

I hope this is clear and easy.

Let us see a calculation-based fill-in-blanks type question.

Example:

A nurse gives 35 mg of meperidine IM q 4 hr prm for pain. The medicine in the ampule marks 50 mg per ml. The volume of medicine that should be given is_____.

The formula to calculate the dose in ml is the desired dose divided by the stock dose multiplied by the medicine label or dilution which gives us 0.7ml.

Dose in ml=(Desired dose/Stock dose) x dilution (med. label) = 35mg/50mg x 1 ml= 0.7 ml

Example:

The doctor orders to infuse 2 liters of normal saline over 48 hours. What is the hourly rate of infusion?

(IV drip in ml/hr)

Round up to the nearest unit figure

Answer:

The order is 2 liters over 48 hours. 2L/48 hr

So converting this into ml/hr, we have

2 x 1000 ml /48hr

41.6ml/hr.

We are asked to round up to the nearest unit figure. So, after rounding up, your answer should be 42 ml/hr.

Strategy to solve fill in the blanks type questions in Next Generation NCLEX RN Exam:

Read the entire question carefully: Before attempting to fill in the blanks, read the entire question to understand the context and identify any clues or hints that may help you select the correct answer.

Identify the missing word: After reading the question, identify the blank and determine what type of word would fit in the blank based on the context of the sentence.

Review the provided options: Next, review the answer choices provided and eliminate any that do not fit the context of the sentence. This can help narrow down your options and increase your chances of selecting the correct answer.

Use your knowledge and critical thinking skills: Apply your knowledge of the subject matter to determine the correct word that would fit in the blank. Additionally, use your critical thinking skills to determine which word would make the most sense in the given sentence.

Double-check your answer: Before submitting your answer, double-check to make sure the word you selected fits grammatically and logically in the sentence.

Case Study: A 65-year-old patient with a history of hypertension and type 2 diabetes mellitus is admitted to the hospital with complaints of shortness of breath and chest pain. Upon examination, the healthcare provider notes an elevated blood pressure of 170/95 mmHg and a blood glucose level of 250 mg/dL.

Question: The healthcare provider should administer _____ to the patient to lower the blood pressure.

A. Insulin
B. Amlodipine
C. Metformin
D. Lisinopril

Strategy:

Read the entire question carefully: In this case, the question asks which medication the healthcare provider should administer to lower the patient's blood pressure.

Identify the missing word: The blank is asking for the name of the medication.

Review the provided options: There are four options given: Insulin, Amlodipine, Metformin, and Lisinopril. Based on the context of the sentence, Insulin and Metformin are unlikely to be the correct options since they are used to treat diabetes, not hypertension.

Use your knowledge and critical thinking skills: Amlodipine and Lisinopril are both medications used to treat hypertension. However, in this case, Lisinopril may be the better option since it is an ACE inhibitor and can also help protect the kidneys, which is important in patients with diabetes.

Double-check your answer: Before submitting your answer, double-check to make sure the word "Lisinopril" fits grammatically and logically in the sentence. The sentence should read: "The healthcare provider should administer Lisinopril to the patient to lower the blood pressure."

Multiple options/Response Questions

This is one of the hardest and most confusing question types in the NCLEX examination. Basically, you may be asked to select all the answers related to nursing management of some condition or any other situations and you have to select all the possible options. Make sure you select all the answers as failure to select one of the correct answers or selecting one wrong and one right answer will make the entire answer wrong.

Example:

A patient is currently in anti-lipid therapy and is given a statin type of drug. Which of the following is a must to follow in this condition?

    i.   Give the drug in the early morning.
    ii. Make sure the patient doesn't consume grapefruit juice during the drug course.
    iii. Make sure the patient is not pregnant.
    iv. Make sure to look for liver enzymes or any hepatic impairment.

The correct answer to this question is options 2, 3, and 4 . option 1 is incorrect. Statins or anti-lipids are basically given at night because most of the cholesterol is synthesized when dietary intake is at lowest.

Option 2 is correct. Grapefruit can block the enzyme to which the drug goes and bind so there will be too much-unbounded drug in the body. The effect of the drug is increased to show side effects so the patient should not be given grapefruit juice.

Option 3 is correct. These drugs are not safe for pregnant women and

Option 4 is also correct because one of the side effect of these drugs is hepatic impairment. So if there is a patient who already has liver problems, this can aggravate the situation. The other side effects of anti-lipids are sore muscles, rhabdomyolysis, arthralgia, dizziness and upper respiratory tract infections.

Rhabdomyolysis is the breakdown of muscle tissue that leads to the release of muscle fiber contents into the blood which affects the kidney and often leads to kidney failure. Arthralgia means stiff joints.

PART I: NCLEX Mastery: Essential Categories and Key Focus Areas for Success

Ethical / Legal aspects/ Professional Standards in Nursing

Here are some key points before entering the practice Question section. Remember, we will study the theoretical concepts more in the explanation part of the practice question. These are just important concepts:

- Administering incorrect medication to a client can lead to adverse consequences, such as allergic reactions, side effects, and interactions with other medications.
- Nurses have a professional and moral obligation to report medication errors to their superiors, irrespective of whether the mistake resulted in harm to the client.
- Failure to report medication errors can result in a nurse facing disciplinary action, legal penalties, and damage to their professional reputation.
- Before performing any surgical or invasive operation, obtaining informed consent is a legal and ethical requirement, and not doing so can result in legal and ethical ramifications for the healthcare provider.
- Informed consent necessitates that the client is thoroughly informed about the proposed procedure's risks, benefits, and alternatives and has the capacity to make an informed decision.
- The privacy and confidentiality of patients are essential rights, and healthcare providers have a moral and legal obligation to safeguard patient information.
- Breaching confidentiality can have legal and ethical implications for healthcare providers, including disciplinary action and harm to their professional reputation.
- Patients have the right to access their medical records and have the information explained to them, as well as the right to give or withhold consent for treatment.
- Honoring a patient's autonomy includes recognizing their right to make informed decisions about their healthcare, even if healthcare providers may not make the same choices for themselves.
- Maintaining accurate documentation is a critical aspect of healthcare since it ensures a complete record of the care provided and aids in maintaining continuity of care.

Beneficence: Focuses on promoting patient well-being by balancing treatment benefits with potential risks to improve health and quality of life.

Fidelity: Involves honoring commitments and promises made to patients, emphasizing trust and reliability in the provider-patient relationship.

Autonomy: Respects a patient's right to make their own healthcare decisions, ensuring their choices and preferences are honored without interference.

Que: Which of the following statements reflects the principle of Beneficence?

A) "It is crucial to respect a patient's right to make their own healthcare decisions."

B) "Healthcare providers must ensure that they do not cause any harm to their patients."

C) "Healthcare providers should strive to promote well-being while balancing benefits and harms, without overriding the patient's preferences."

D) "The duty to tell the truth and be transparent with patients is fundamental."

Correct Answer: C

Explanation:

Option A describes Autonomy, which focuses on respecting a person's right to make their own choices.

Option B describes Nonmaleficence, which emphasizes avoiding harm to others.

Option C is correct because it outlines Beneficence, which involves promoting well-being and carefully weighing benefits and harms, while also noting the issue of paternalism.

Option D describes Veracity, which concerns truthfulness and transparency.

> **tip** **When obtaining informed consent for medical procedures, ensure that patients are fully informed about the risks, benefits, and alternatives. Engage in thorough verbal explanations, answer Question, and provide written materials to support understanding. Avoid requesting signatures on consent forms without prior discussion, as this may violate the patient's right to make an informed decision about their healthcare.**

Que: Which situations could compromise a client's privacy?

A. Leaving a confused client in a public hallway

B. Interviewing a client with a solid wall separating them from others

C. Allowing unauthorized individuals to observe a procedure

D. Using a client's photo on the healthcare facility's website with their consent

E. Discussing a client's medical condition in a private, secure office

Correct Answers: A and C

Explanation:

A (Correct): Leaving a confused client in a public hallway compromises their privacy by exposing them to public view and potential discomfort.

B (Incorrect): Interviewing a client with a solid wall separating them from others ensures privacy and is not a privacy breach.

C (Correct): Allowing unauthorized individuals to observe a procedure without the client's consent breaches their privacy by exposing their treatment to others.

D (Incorrect): Using a client's photo on the healthcare facility's website with their consent is appropriate and does not violate privacy.

E (Incorrect): Discussing a client's medical condition in a private, secure office upholds privacy by ensuring that the conversation is confidential.

Mark is scheduled for surgery at the hospital. He's expressed concerns about understanding the surgery's risks and benefits before consenting. The healthcare provider presents him with a consent form. Which of the following actions by the healthcare provider would violate Mark's right to informed consent?

A. Thoroughly explaining the surgery's potential risks and benefits, and answering all of Mark's Question before seeking his consent.

B. Requesting Mark's signature on the consent form without providing any information about the surgery or its potential consequences.

C. Briefly explaining the surgery's risks without discussing its potential benefits or alternatives.

D. Providing Mark with written information about the surgery but not discussing it verbally before seeking his consent.

Explanation:

Option B is correct as it violates Mark's right to informed consent. Informed consent necessitates Mark being fully informed about the surgery's risks, benefits, and alternatives. Requesting Mark to sign the consent form without providing any information about the surgery or its potential consequences fails to meet this requirement, thus violating his right to make an informed decision about his healthcare.

Option A is incorrect as it represents the appropriate approach, providing detailed information and answering question before seeking consent.

Option C is incorrect as it only addresses risks and not benefits or alternatives, which falls short of a comprehensive informed consent process.

Option D is incorrect as providing written information is commendable, but it should be accompanied by verbal explanation and discussion with the patient to ensure their understanding and informed decision-making.

Que: Which of the following is NOT typically included in a medication prescription?

A. Date and time prescription was written

B. Patient's social security number

C. Medication name

D. Route of administration

E. Healthcare provider's signature

Answer-Not Typically included: B

Explanation:

- A (Incorrect): The date and time when the prescription was written are essential components of a medication prescription to ensure proper timing and validity.
- B (Correct): The patient's social security number is not typically included in a medication prescription. Prescriptions usually do not require this level of personal identification.
- C (Incorrect): The medication name is a critical component of a prescription, indicating what drug is being prescribed.
- D (Incorrect): The route of administration specifies how the medication should be taken (e.g., orally, intravenously) and is an essential part of the prescription.
- E (Incorrect): The healthcare provider's signature is necessary to validate and authorize the prescription.

> **tip** When documenting patient care, prioritize accuracy and professionalism. Use a black ink pen for legibility and ensure timely documentation to maintain complete and accurate records. Document client responses to interventions as it is crucial for tracking progress. Minimize the use of abbreviations to avoid errors and misunderstandings. Never leave blank spaces on documentation forms, and follow agency policies for making corrections to errors.

Que: A nurse, experiencing pressure and stress due to a heavy workload, is responsible for documenting patient care at the hospital. However, during this stressful situation, the nurse unintentionally neglects to document a medication administration.

Which of the following statements made by the nurse accurately reflects appropriate documentation guidelines?

A) It's preferable to use a black ink pen for narrative documentation to ensure legibility and professionalism.

B) Timely documentation of care, medications, treatments, and procedures is not essential.

C) Documenting client responses to interventions is an optional practice.

D) Documentation should mainly consist of subjective data.

E) Employing as many abbreviations as possible is encouraged for time-saving.

F) Leaving blank spaces on documentation forms is permissible.

G) Corrections for documentation errors should be made by erasing and rewriting the information.

The correct answer is A.

> **tip** When documenting patient care, use black ink for professionalism, ensure timely and objective notes, avoid excessive abbreviations, and follow proper correction procedures without leaving blank spaces.

A) Using a black ink pen for narrative documentation ensures legibility and professionalism, which is essential for accurate records.

B) Timely documentation is crucial for maintaining a complete and accurate record of patient care, making option B incorrect.

C) Documenting client responses is vital to track progress and adjust care plans accordingly, making option C incorrect.

D) Documentation should primarily consist of objective, factual, and comprehensive information, making option D incorrect.

E) While abbreviations can save time, using too many may lead to errors and misunderstandings, making option E incorrect.

F) Leaving blank spaces on documentation forms may be seen as incomplete and unprofessional, making option F incorrect.

G) Corrections for documentation errors should be made following agency policies, which may include striking through the error, initialing, and dating it, rather than erasing and rewriting information, making option G incorrect.

The nurse providing preoperative care explains the procedure and its risks and benefits to Mrs. Alvin and obtains her surgical consent. However, on the day of the surgery, Mrs. Alvin expresses doubts about the surgery and question if it is really necessary.

Which of the following statements from Mrs. Alvin indicates that the nurse did not obtain an informed consent for the surgery?

A. "I have discussed the surgery with my family, and they support my decision."

B. "I am not sure if I really need this surgery."

C. "I am excited to have the surgery and get back to my normal activities."

D. "I am worried about the anesthesia, but I trust my surgeon."

E. "I have signed the consent form, but I don't know what it says."

F. "I understand that there are risks involved in the surgery, but I trust my healthcare team."

G. "I believe this surgery is the best option for me."

Answers : B, E, G

> **tip** Informed consent is a legal and ethical requirement for all surgical or invasive procedures. The consent form documents that the client has been informed of the risks, benefits, and possible alternatives to the proposed procedure.

In this case, the following statements from Mrs. Alvin indicate that she may not have fully understood the risks and benefits of the procedure, and therefore, the nurse may not have obtained an informed consent from her:

Option B because it shows Mrs. Alvin's uncertainty about the necessity of the surgery.

Option E because it indicates that Mrs. Alvin signed the consent form without understanding its contents.

Option G because it suggests a lack of clarity regarding the necessity of the surgery.

Que: Which of the following statements made by a client is a valid right statement?

1. "I can expect the hospital to provide every possible type of health service, no matter their specific focus or limitations."

2. "I have the right to be informed about my diagnosis, possible treatment options, and the likely outcomes, and to discuss this information with my healthcare provider."

3. "I can refuse treatment without needing to be informed about the potential consequences of my decision."

4. "I have the right to examine my medical records and receive explanations about the details contained in them."

5. "I am entitled to know if the hospital has any affiliations with external organizations that might affect my care or treatment."

Explanation of Options:

1. **"I can expect the hospital to provide every possible type of health service, no matter their specific focus or limitations."**: This is incorrect. Although patients have a right to necessary health services, it's unrealistic to expect all possible services from any hospital. Hospitals have specific scopes of practice and resource limitations.

2. **"I have the right to be informed about my diagnosis, possible treatment options, and the likely outcomes, and to discuss this information with my healthcare provider."**: This is correct. Clients have the right to detailed information about their diagnosis and treatment options and to discuss these with their healthcare provider to make informed decisions.

3. **"I can refuse treatment without needing to be informed about the potential consequences of my decision."**: This is incorrect. While clients do have the right to refuse treatment, they must also be informed about the possible consequences of their refusal to make an informed decision.

4. **"I have the right to examine my medical records and receive explanations about the details contained in them."**: This is correct. Patients have the right to access their medical records and to have any unclear information explained to them.

5. **"I am entitled to know if the hospital has any affiliations with external organizations that might affect my care or treatment."**: This is correct. Clients should be informed about any external relationships the hospital has that could impact their care or treatment decisions.

Que : Which case study is not relevant for maintaining patient confidentiality in nursing practice?

Case Study 1:

A: Nurse Taylor, who is working the night shift in a busy hospital, discusses a patient's treatment plan with a colleague from another unit in the hospital's shared break room. The conversation includes detailed information about the patient's diagnosis and ongoing treatment. Other hospital staff who are not involved in the patient's care overhear the discussion.

Case Study 2:

B: Nurse Johnson is reviewing a patient's medical records on a hospital computer in a private office. The door is closed, and the computer is secured with a password. Nurse Johnson ensures that no unauthorized personnel have access to the patient's information and that any conversations about the patient's case are conducted discreetly within the office.

Case Study 3:

C: Nurse Anderson is excited about a patient's successful recovery and posts an update about the patient's condition on her personal social media account. The post includes details about the patient's progress and some specific health information. Nurse Anderson did not obtain consent from the patient before sharing this information online.

Case Study 4:

D: Nurse Lee is meeting with a patient's family to discuss the patient's care plan. The meeting is held in a designated conference room within the hospital where only the patient's family and Nurse Lee are present. Nurse Lee ensures that the conversation is conducted privately and that no sensitive information is overheard by unauthorized individuals.

Options:

A. Case Study 1

B. Case Study 2

C. Case Study 3

D. Case Study 4

Explanation of Options:

A. Case Study 1: Incorrect. Discussing a patient's treatment plan with a colleague who is not involved in the patient's care in a public area like the break room breaches confidentiality. Such discussions should be restricted to private and secure settings with only those involved in the patient's care.

B. Case Study 2: Correct. Reviewing patient information in a private office with secured access and ensuring no unauthorized individuals have access to the information adheres to confidentiality practices. It ensures the privacy and security of patient information.

C. Case Study 3: Incorrect. Posting details about a patient's condition on a personal social media account without the patient's consent is a violation of patient confidentiality. Information about patients should remain confidential and should not be shared publicly or without explicit consent.

D. Case Study 4: Correct. Discussing the patient's care plan with the family in a private conference room, with only authorized individuals present, maintains patient confidentiality. This practice ensures that sensitive information is shared appropriately and privately.

Que :

Case Study 1:

A: Nurse Smith takes a photograph of a patient receiving treatment to share with her colleagues, hoping to use it for educational purposes. The photograph includes identifiable features of the patient.

Case Study 2:

B: Nurse Brown discusses a patient's medical condition with a family member in the hospital lobby. The family member is not authorized to receive this information, and the discussion is overheard by others.

Case Study 3:

C: Nurse Lee interviews a patient in a private room with only a curtain separating them from another patient. The conversation about the patient's treatment is clearly audible to the other patient and visitors.

Case Study 4:

D: Nurse Taylor leaves the room door open while performing a procedure on a patient, allowing anyone passing by to see the treatment being administered.

E: Nurse Lee meets with a patient's family in a private conference room to discuss the patient's care plan. Only the family and Nurse Lee are present.

Que : Which case study demonstrates a violation of client privacy?

Options:

A. Case Study 1

B. Case Study 2

C. Case Study 3

D. Case Study 4

Explanation of Options:

A. Case Study 1: Incorrect. Taking photographs of a patient without their consent is a violation of privacy. This action includes identifiable features of the patient and is not allowed without explicit permission from the patient.

B. Case Study 2: Incorrect. Discussing a patient's medical condition with an unauthorized person in a public area breaches confidentiality .

C. Case Study 3: Incorrect. Interviewing a patient in a room with a curtain separating them from another patient violates privacy in terms of confidentiality.

D. Case Study 4: Incorrect. Leaving the door open during a procedure violates privacy as it allows others to view the treatment.

Positioning of the patient

- Proper positioning of clients is important for their comfort and recovery, and to prevent complications such as pressure ulcers.
- Different bed positions, such as flat-bed, Fowler's position, Trendelenburg's position, prone position, and sitting position, are used depending on the patient's condition and the procedure being performed.
- The position of choice for patients with respiratory distress syndrome is Fowler's position, which allows for better lung expansion and ease in breathing.
- Trendelenburg's position is used during lower abdominal surgeries, central venous catheter placement, and to treat low cardiac output, but should not be used in lung disorders.
- Reverse Trendelenburg's position is used to prevent esophageal reflux and orthostatic hypotension.
- Prone position is helpful for patients requiring a breathing machine, full extension of hip and knees, and better lung drainage in certain lung conditions, but should not be used for patients with spine surgery or spine problems.
- Sitting position is suitable for people who have difficulty in breathing and exhaling.
- Lithotomy position is common for childbirth and vaginal examination.
- Keeping the leg elevated above the level of heart is helpful for patients with varicose veins.

Que: Patient Information: Kurrim is a 65-year-old male admitted to the hospital for lower abdominal surgery. He has a history of hypertension and is currently experiencing hypotension. The surgical procedure requires a Trendelenburg position. As a nurse, you need to ensure the proper positioning of Kurrim to maintain his comfort, safety, and overall well-being.

Scenario: Kurrim is scheduled for lower abdominal surgery due to a medical condition. The surgical team has determined that the Trendelenburg position is necessary for this procedure due to his hypotension. As a nurse, you need to understand the principles of proper patient positioning and provide appropriate care for Kurrim during the surgery.

Que : Which patient positioning would be appropriate for Kurrim during his lower abdominal surgery due to hypotension?

A) Supine position

B) Fowler's position

C) Trendelenburg's position

D) Semi-Fowler's position

E) Prone position

F) Lateral decubitus position

G) Sims position H) Lithotomy position

Correct Answer: C) Trendelenburg's position

Explanation: Trendelenburg's position is appropriate for patients with hypotension because it helps improve blood circulation to vital organs. In this position, the patient's head is lower than their feet, which assists in increasing venous return to the heart and can help raise blood pressure. This is particularly useful in cases of shock and hypotension, as seen in Kurrim's case.
Let's discuss why other options are incorrect:
A) Supine position: This is the standard position where the patient lies flat on their back. It's commonly used for many types of surgeries.
B) Fowler's position: Fowler's position is typically used for patients with respiratory distress and cardiovascular issues, not for hypotension.
D) Semi-Fowler's position: Semi-Fowler's position is similar to Fowler's position and is not indicated for hypotension.
E) Prone position: The prone position is not recommended for patients with respiratory or cardiovascular issues, which makes it unsuitable for Kurrim.
F) Lateral decubitus position: This position is used for patients with respiratory distress or pressure sore prevention but is not indicated for hypotension.
G) Sims position: The Sims position is used for rectal examinations or enema administration, which is not relevant to Kurrim's condition.
H) Lithotomy position: Lithotomy position is used for gynecological or urological procedures, and it is not suitable for hypotension during abdominal surgery.

A nurse is preparing a female patient, Maria, for a medical procedure that requires specific positioning. Maria is scheduled for a gynecological exam due to persistent pelvic pain and is anxious about the process. The nurse must decide the best position for Maria to ensure proper access for the examination while maintaining her comfort and safety.

Question

Which of the following positions is most appropriate for Maria's gynecological exam?

A) Fowler's position
B) Lateral decubitus position
C) Supine position
D) Lithotomy position
E) Prone position

Nurse's Statements in Options:

1. **Option A (Fowler's position) - Incorrect**

- Nurse's statement: "I believe Fowler's position will help Maria feel more comfortable since it involves a semi-upright posture."
- **Explanation**: Fowler's position is used to support patients with respiratory or cardiovascular issues and is not suitable for gynecological exams. It would not provide adequate access for the pelvic area.

2. **Option B (Lateral decubitus position) - Incorrect**
   - Nurse's statement: "This position could be helpful for reducing pressure on certain parts of the body, but it doesn't provide good access for a pelvic examination."
   - **Explanation**: Lateral decubitus is primarily used for pressure sore prevention or to facilitate respiratory function. It does not offer sufficient access for a gynecological examination.

3. **Option C (Supine position) - Incorrect**
   - Nurse's statement: "Maria could lie flat on her back for comfort, but this may not provide enough visibility for the gynecological exam."
   - **Explanation**: The supine position does not provide optimal leg positioning and access for procedures like a gynecological examination.

4. **Option D (Lithotomy position) - Correct**
   - Nurse's statement: "For Maria's gynecological exam, the lithotomy position is the best choice as it allows optimal access to the pelvic area."
   - **Explanation**: The lithotomy position, where the patient lies on her back with her legs elevated and supported by stirrups, is specifically designed for procedures like gynecological exams, childbirth, or urological procedures, making it the correct choice.

5. **Option E (Prone position) - Incorrect**
   - Nurse's statement: "Perhaps the prone position could be useful for back procedures, but it won't be effective for Maria's pelvic exam."
   - **Explanation**: The prone position involves lying on the stomach and is not suitable for any kind of pelvic examination or procedure involving the front of the body.

Correct Answer: D (Lithotomy position). The lithotomy position is the most appropriate for gynecological exams as it provides the necessary access to the pelvic area, ensuring both safety and effectiveness during the procedure.

Que: The nurse is preparing to position a patient experiencing difficulty breathing. The patient's condition requires that they be placed in a position that promotes lung expansion and reduces respiratory distress. The nurse correctly chooses _____ position, which involves the patient's head being elevated to approximately _____ degrees.

A) Prone; 0

B) Fowler's; 45-60

C) Supine; 180

D) Trendelenburg's; 30

E) Lithotomy; 90

Correct Answer:

B) Fowler's; 45-60

Explanation:

Option A (Prone; 0) - Incorrect

Reasoning: The prone position involves lying flat on the stomach, which does not aid in respiratory distress as it can impede lung expansion. Additionally, "0 degrees" does not fit the description for elevating the head.

Option B (Fowler's; 45-60) - Correct

Reasoning: Fowler's position involves elevating the patient's head to 45-60 degrees, which helps with lung expansion and alleviates respiratory issues. It is the best choice for patients with difficulty breathing.

Option C (Supine; 180) - Incorrect

Reasoning: The supine position involves lying flat on the back, typically at 180 degrees. This position does not provide head elevation and is not effective for promoting lung expansion in patients with respiratory distress.

Option D (Trendelenburg's; 30) - Incorrect

Reasoning: Trendelenburg's position involves the patient's head being lower than the feet, which is not suitable for promoting lung expansion or improving breathing. The 30-degree angle refers to the tilt rather than elevation of the head.

Option E (Lithotomy; 90) - Incorrect

Reasoning: The lithotomy position is used primarily for gynecological or urological procedures. A "90-degree" elevation refers to the patient's legs, not the head, making it inappropriate for patients with respiratory problems.

Correct Answer: B (Fowler's; 45-60). Fowler's position, with the head elevated to 45-60 degrees, is most suitable for improving lung expansion and reducing respiratory distress.

Total Parenteral Nutrition

Total Parenteral Nutrition (TPN) is a critical method of providing nutrition to patients unable to intake food via their gastrointestinal tract, offering a customized solution tailored to individual needs. It replenishes calories, restores nitrogen balance, and replaces essential fluids, vitamins, electrolytes, minerals, and trace elements. Administered intravenously, TPN, also known as IV nutrition feeding, necessitates understanding its composition, which varies based on factors like age and organ function. Components typically include water, energy, amino acids, essential fatty acids, vitamins, and minerals, with lipid emulsions occasionally included.

To administer TPN effectively, nurses must comprehend its indications, limitations, and associated risks. Vigilant monitoring of patients receiving TPN is crucial, encompassing fluid and electrolyte status, blood glucose levels, liver and kidney function tests, and skin integrity changes. Awareness of potential complications, such as fat embolism in patients with pulmonary edema, and management of electrolyte imbalances and acid-base disturbances are paramount. Proper administration techniques, including aseptic practices, infusion pump management, and adherence to facility policies, ensure patient safety and optimal outcomes in TPN therapy.

Furthermore, interventions like monitoring albumin levels and avoiding medication additions to the TPN solution during infusion contribute to effective patient management. Clients undergoing TPN therapy require close monitoring for weight gain and fluid retention, with adjustments made to optimize nutritional support and minimize complications. TPN is administered into a vein, generally through a PICC line or a central line due to its hypertonic nature, which can cause vein irritation. Clients ideally gain 0.5 to 1 kg/week on TPN, with weight gain exceeding 0.5 kg/day indicating fluid retention. It's critical to infuse or discard any TPN solution within 24 hours once the administration set is attached, and never add medications to a TPN solution container once it's actively infusing. Additionally, excess amino acid intake on TPN therapy should prompt monitoring of blood urea nitrogen and creatinine levels. Understanding these facets of TPN therapy is essential for nurses managing patients requiring this specialized nutritional intervention.

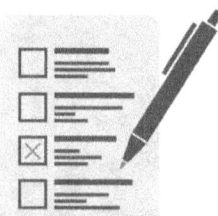

Practice Session

Que : Nurse Rynki is caring for a patient who has been receiving TPN for the past week. The patient has been experiencing abdominal cramps, lethargy, confusion, malaise, muscle weakness, and tetany. Rynki checks the patient's electrolyte levels and finds that they are imbalanced.

What should Nurse Rynki do to address the patient's electrolyte imbalance?

A) Administer medications to the patient's TPN solution

B) Discard the TPN solution and start a new one

C) Administer electrolyte supplements to the patient

D) Increase the rate of TPN infusion

Correct Answer: C

Strategy to Solve the Problem:

Nurse Rynki should consider the patient's symptoms and the fact that TPN can cause electrolyte imbalances. She should also consider the fact that adding medications to the TPN solution or increasing the rate of infusion would not address the patient's electrolyte imbalance. The best option to address the imbalance is to administer electrolyte supplements to the patient.

Option A is incorrect because it is not recommended to add medications to a TPN solution once it is actively infusing. Option B is incorrect because discarding the TPN solution would not address the patient's electrolyte imbalance. Option D is incorrect because increasing the rate of TPN infusion would not address the electrolyte imbalance and could potentially cause further problems. Option C is the correct answer because electrolyte supplements can help restore the balance of electrolytes in the patient's body.

Que : A patient, Mary, is admitted to the hospital with severe gastrointestinal issues that prevent her from receiving nutrition orally. She has been prescribed TPN as a means of providing her with the necessary nutrients. As a registered nurse, you are responsible for administering the TPN to Mary.

Which of the following is NOT an ingredient in TPN solutions?

a) Water

b) Energy

c) Amino acids

d) Insulin

Correct answer: d) Insulin

TPN solutions are designed to provide the body with the necessary nutrients that it cannot obtain through oral intake. This includes things like water, energy, amino acids, essential fatty acids, vitamins, minerals, and trace elements. Insulin is not a necessary nutrient for the body, but rather a hormone that helps regulate blood sugar levels. Therefore, it is not typically included in TPN solutions.

Option a) Water is a necessary ingredient in TPN solutions as it helps to provide hydration and support the body's various functions. Option b) Energy, in the form of calories, is also an important component of

TPN as it helps to provide the body with the fuel it needs to function. Option c) Amino acids are essential for the body's growth and repair, and are therefore included in TPN solutions. Option d) Insulin is not typically an ingredient in TPN solutions, as it is a hormone that helps regulate blood sugar levels and is not a necessary nutrient for the body. Therefore, the correct answer is d) Insulin.

Mrs. Gunjan is a 58 year old patient who has been admitted to the hospital for malnutrition. She has been experiencing difficulty swallowing due to an esophageal stricture and has not been able to maintain a healthy diet. The doctor has decided to initiate TPN as a means of providing nutrition for Mrs. Gunjan. As a registered nurse, you will be responsible for administering the TPN and monitoring Mrs. Gunjan's progress.

What should be considered when administering TPN to a patient with altered fat metabolism or conditions that disrupt normal fat metabolism?

A) The TPN should be administered through a PICC line.
B) The patient should be monitored for signs of electrolyte imbalance.
C) The TPN should not be administered.
D) The patient's protein levels should be checked.

Correct Answer: C) The TPN should not be administered.

To solve this problem, the nurse must be familiar with the contraindications for TPN administration. In this case, the patient has altered fat metabolism or conditions that disrupt normal fat metabolism, which is a contraindication for TPN administration.
Rationale and Explanation:

Option A) is incorrect because the type of access used for TPN administration does not affect the contraindications for TPN.

Option B) is incorrect because electrolyte imbalances are a potential complication of TPN, but are not a contraindication for its use.

Option D) is incorrect because protein levels may drop initially in a patient receiving TPN, but this is not a contraindication for its use.

Option C) is the correct answer because TPN should not be administered to patients with altered fat metabolism or conditions that disrupt normal fat metabolism. This is because TPN contains essential fatty acids and lipid emulsions, which can exacerbate these conditions and potentially cause harm to the patient.

Blood and Blood Products

> Compatibility of blood transfusion is very important to check before administering it to the patient.
> As a nurse, you should match the name of the patient with the identification band and label on the blood sample.
> Before transfusion, the Rh and Blood Group Type (ABO) should be assessed.
> Blood grouping classifies blood based on the inherited properties of red blood cells (erythrocytes) as determined by the presence or absence of the antigens A and B.
> In Rh factor, the protein found on the surface of red blood cells is inherited and is either positive or negative.
> Compatibility is checked with crossmatching where donor's RBCs are combined with the serum of recipient.
> Donors of type A can transfuse blood to recipients of type A and type AB blood group, donors of type B can transfuse blood to recipients of type B and AB, and donors of type AB can transfuse blood to recipients of type AB.
> Donors of type O can transfuse blood to recipients of type A, type B, type AB, and type O, making it the universal donor.
> Recipients of type AB can receive blood from all donors, making it the universal recipient.
> Rh negative clients should never be transfused blood from Rh positive donors.

Blood Group	Can Receive Blood From	Can Donate Blood To
A+	A+, A-, O+, O-	A+, AB+
A-	A-, O-	A+, A-, AB+, AB-
B+	B+, B-, O+, O-	B+, AB+
B-	B-, O-	B+, B-, AB+, AB-
AB+	All blood types	AB+
AB-	AB-, A-, B-, O-	AB+, AB-
O+	O+, O-	A+, B+, AB+, O+
O-	O-	A+, A-, B+, B-, AB+, AB-

Que: Which blood type can receive from any Rh-positive blood type?

A) O-

B) A-

C) B+

D) AB+

E) A+

Correct Answer: E) A+

Explanation:

A) O-: Incorrect. O- blood can only receive from O- blood.

B) A-: Incorrect. A- blood can receive from A-, A+, O-, and O+ blood, but not Rh-positive.

C) B+: Incorrect. B+ blood can receive from B+, B-, O+, and O- blood.

D) AB+: Incorrect. AB+ blood can receive from all blood types, not just Rh-positive.

E) A+: Correct. A+ blood can receive from A+, A-, O+, and O- blood, including Rh-positive.

Que: Which blood type is a universal recipient and can receive blood from all other types?

A) A-

B) B+

C) AB-

D) AB+

E) O-

Correct Answer: D) AB+

Explanation:

A) A-: Incorrect. A- can receive from A-, A+, O-, and O+ blood.

B) B+: Incorrect. B+ can receive from B+, B-, O+, and O- blood.

C) AB-: Incorrect. AB- can receive from AB-, AB+, A-, A+, B-, B+, O-, and O+ blood but not O+.

D) AB+: Correct. AB+ is the universal recipient and can receive from all blood types.

E) O-: Incorrect. O- is the universal donor but not a universal recipient.

Que: Which of the following blood types can only donate to AB+ recipients?

A) B+

B) O+

C) A-

D) AB-

E) AB+

Correct Answer: E) AB+

Explanation:

A) B+: Incorrect. B+ can donate to B+ and AB+.

B) O+: Incorrect. O+ can donate to O+, A+, B+, and AB+.

C) A-: Incorrect. A- can donate to A-, A+, AB-, and AB+.

D) AB-: Incorrect. AB- can donate to AB- and AB+.

E) AB+: Correct. AB+ can only donate to AB+.

 NGN Case Study

Patient History:
Patient Name: Kurrim Smith Age: 45 Gender: Male Medical Record Number: 123456 Admission Date: September 1, 2023
Chief Complaint:
Kurrim Smith, a 45-year-old male, was admitted to the hospital with a diagnosis of severe anemia due to chronic gastrointestinal bleeding. He presents with fatigue, shortness of breath, and dizziness. The patient's medical history includes a previous episode of peptic ulcer disease and a family history of anemia.
Vital Signs:
• Blood Pressure: 110/70 mmHg
• Heart Rate: 90 beats per minute
• Respiratory Rate: 18 breaths per minute
• Temperature: 98.6°F (37°C)
• Oxygen Saturation: 94% on room air
Laboratory Values:
• Hemoglobin (Hb): 7.2 g/dL (Normal range: 12-16 g/dL)

- Hematocrit (Hct): 24% (Normal range: 36-48%)
- Red Blood Cell Count (RBC): 2.5 million/mm³ (Normal range: 4.5-5.5 million/mm³)
- Blood Type: A positive (ABO) and Rh positive
- Serum Bilirubin: 1.0 mg/dL (Normal range: 0.2-1.2 mg/dL)

Medical History:

Kurrim has a history of chronic gastrointestinal bleeding, which has led to severe anemia. He has been receiving iron supplements and other conservative treatments for the past six months, but his condition has not improved significantly.

Social History:

Kurrim is a non-smoker and consumes alcohol occasionally. He has a sedentary lifestyle and a family history of anemia, with his mother and maternal grandmother both having been diagnosed with iron-deficiency anemia.

Current Medications:
- Iron supplements
- Pantoprazole (for gastric acid suppression)

Que: Which blood type can Kurrim Smith, a patient with A positive (ABO) and Rh positive blood type, receive a transfusion from without risk of compatibility issues?

A) Type A positive

B) Type B positive

C) Type AB positive

D) Type O positive

E) Type O negative

Kurrim Smith's blood type is A positive (A+). This means he has:

A antigens on the surface of his red blood cells.

Rh factor (a protein) on the surface of his red blood cells.

Anti-B antibodies in his plasma.

Compatible Blood Types

Type A positive (A+):

A antigens: Matches Kurrim's A antigens.

Rh factor: Matches Kurrim's Rh positive status.

Anti-B antibodies: Not present in the donor blood, so no reaction with Kurrim's blood.

Type O positive (O+):

No A or B antigens: Safe because there are no antigens to react with Kurrim's anti-B antibodies.

Rh factor: Matches Kurrim's Rh positive status.

Anti-A and Anti-B antibodies: Present in the donor plasma, but since the red blood cells are transfused without significant plasma, this is generally safe.

Type O negative (O-):

No A or B antigens: Safe because there are no antigens to react with Kurrim's anti-B antibodies.

No Rh factor: Safe because it won't react with Kurrim's Rh positive status.

Anti-A and Anti-B antibodies: Present in the donor plasma, but since the red blood cells are transfused without significant plasma, this is generally safe.

Incompatible Blood Types

Type B positive (B+):

B antigens: Would react with Kurrim's anti-B antibodies, causing a dangerous immune response.

Type AB positive (AB+):

A and B antigens: The B antigens would react with Kurrim's anti-B antibodies, causing a dangerous immune response.

Summary

Kurrim can safely receive blood from:

Type A positive (A+)

Type O positive (O+)

Type O negative (O-)

These types are compatible because they either match his antigens and Rh factor or lack the antigens that would cause an immune response.

> **tip** Ensuring the compatibility of blood transfusion is paramount in patient care. As a nurse, it is imperative to meticulously match the patient's name with the identification band and label on the blood sample. Before administering a transfusion, assessing the Rh factor and Blood Group Type (ABO) is crucial. Blood grouping categorizes blood based on the presence or absence of antigens A and B on red blood cells. The Rh factor, either positive or negative, determines the protein found on the surface of red blood cells and is inherited. Compatibility is verified through crossmatching, where donor red blood cells are combined with the recipient's serum. Type A donors can provide blood to recipients with type A and AB blood groups, while type B donors can supply blood to recipients with type B and AB. Type AB donors are compatible with recipients of type AB blood, and type O donors, being the universal donors, can provide blood to recipients of types A, B, AB, and O. Conversely, type AB recipients can receive blood from any donor, making them the universal recipients. Rh negative clients should never receive blood from Rh positive donors. Transfusion complications will be covered in subsequent lectures, underscoring the critical importance of meticulous compatibility checks in blood transfusion procedures.

Blood Components

Packed Red Blood Cells (PRBCs):

Use: Replaces erythrocytes, increases oxygen transport.

Indications: Acute hemorrhage, surgery, oxygen shortage.

Transfusion time: Up to 4 hours.

Platelets:

Use: Clot formation, controls bleeding.

Indications: Thrombocytopenia, cancer therapy, autoimmune diseases.

Fresh Frozen Plasma:

Use: Provides clotting factors, increases blood volume.

Indications: Hypovolemia, shock.

Albumin:

Use: Expands blood volume, replaces plasma proteins.

Cryoprecipitates:

Use: Replaces clotting factors (fibrinogen, factor VIII).

Indications: Hemophilia A, von Willebrand disease.

Whole Blood:

Use: Contains all blood components, used in severe hemorrhage.

Granulocytes:

Use: Treats infections in septic or neutropenic patients unresponsive to antibiotics.

Nursing Considerations:

- Check for transfusion reactions (fever, chills, rash, dyspnea).
- Monitor vital signs before, during, and after transfusion.
- Watch for signs of fluid overload and bleeding.

Blood Transfusion Complications:

Transfusion Reactions:

Types: Hemolytic, allergic, febrile, bacterial.

Symptoms: Chills, fever, rapid pulse, nausea, cough, muscle ache.

Septicemia:

Contaminated blood causing fever, vomiting, diarrhea, hypotension.

Circulatory Overload:

Excess volume leading to tachycardia, chest pain, wheezing.

Iron Overload:

Seen in multiple transfusions; treat with IV deferoxamine.

Disease Transmission:

Risks include Hepatitis C, HIV, malaria.

Citrate Toxicity:

Caused by multiple transfusions leading to hypocalcemia, hypomagnesemia.

Electrolyte Imbalance:

Blood transfusion can cause hypocalcemia or hyperkalemia.

Que: Which action is NOT recommended when administering blood transfusions?

A) Mixing blood with normal saline

B) Adding medications to the blood transfusion

C) Replacing the blood administration set with each unit

D) Checking the blood bag for leaks and abnormalities

E) Ensuring blood is administered within the maximum allowable time frame

Correct Answer: B) Adding medications to the blood transfusion

Explanation:

A) Mixing blood with normal saline: Incorrect. Normal saline is the only solution recommended for mixing with blood components.

B) Adding medications to the blood transfusion: Correct. Medications should never be added to blood components or mixed with blood transfusions.

C) Replacing the blood administration set with each unit: Incorrect. This is a recommended practice to reduce the risk of infection.

D) Checking the blood bag for leaks and abnormalities: Incorrect. This is an essential step to ensure the blood is safe for transfusion.

E) Ensuring blood is administered within the maximum allowable time frame: Incorrect. This is important for maintaining the safety and efficacy of the transfusion.

Que: Who must verify the HCP's prescription, client identity, and blood component tag before a transfusion?

A) The attending physician

B) The blood bank technician

C) Two licensed nurses

D) The patient's family member

E) The hospital administrator

Correct Answer: C) Two licensed nurses

Explanation:

A) The attending physician: Incorrect. While the physician prescribes the blood, the verification of identity and compatibility is not their responsibility.

B) The blood bank technician: Incorrect. The blood bank technician handles the preparation but does not perform bedside verification.

C) Two licensed nurses: Correct. Two licensed nurses must verify the HCP's prescription, client identity, and blood component tag according to agency policy.

D) The patient's family member: Incorrect. Family members are not authorized to perform these verifications.

E) The hospital administrator: Incorrect. The hospital administrator is not involved in the direct process of blood transfusion verification.

Medication Administration

Nurse Monika is preparing medication for a patient. She reads the medication label but miscalculates the dose and administers an incorrect amount. The patient experiences adverse effects from the incorrect dose.

Which of the following statements made by Nurse Monika indicates she does not understand the importance of proper medication administration?

"I'll just give this dose and hope it's correct since I'm running out of time."

"I should monitor the patient's vital signs after administering this medication."

"I'm not sure if this medication needs to be administered with food or on an empty stomach."

"I always check the medication label before administering it to ensure accuracy."

"I need to report any changes in the patient's condition to the healthcare provider."

"I'm going to double-check the patient's chart to make sure the dose is correct."

"I forgot to use sterile technique while preparing this medication."

Answers:

The incorrect options and hence the answer to the question are:

"I'll just give this dose and hope it's correct since I'm running out of time."

"I'm not sure if this medication needs to be administered with food or on an empty stomach."

Explanation:

1. "I'll just give this dose and hope it's correct since I'm running out of time.": This statement shows a lack of understanding of the importance of verifying medication doses and reflects negligence due to rushing. Proper medication administration requires accuracy and cannot be compromised by time constraints.

3. "I'm not sure if this medication needs to be administered with food or on an empty stomach.": This statement indicates a lack of knowledge about the medication's administration requirements, which is crucial for its effectiveness and safety.

Incorrect Options:

2. "I should monitor the patient's vital signs after administering this medication.": This statement shows an understanding of the need to monitor the patient after medication administration, which is a correct practice.

4. "I always check the medication label before administering it to ensure accuracy.": This statement demonstrates proper knowledge and practice in verifying medication before administration.

5. "I need to report any changes in the patient's condition to the healthcare provider.": This statement shows an understanding of the importance of communication regarding patient condition changes.

6. "I'm going to double-check the patient's chart to make sure the dose is correct.": This statement reflects proper practice in verifying medication doses, indicating knowledge and attention to detail.

7. "I forgot to use sterile technique while preparing this medication.": While this statement shows a lapse in technique, it is not directly related to medication administration errors due to dosing inaccuracies.

Que: A patient with cardiovascular concerns is seeking natural remedies to support their condition. Which of the following herbal supplements is most appropriate for helping to lower cholesterol levels?

A. Echinacea

B. Garlic

C. Ginkgo biloba

D. Chamomile

Correct Answer: Garlic

Explanation of Options:

A. Echinacea: Incorrect. Echinacea is known for stimulating the immune system and is not used to lower cholesterol levels. It is more commonly used to support the immune system during colds and infections.

B. Garlic: Correct. Garlic has antioxidant properties and is specifically noted for its use in lowering cholesterol levels. This makes it relevant for cardiovascular health, particularly in managing cholesterol levels, which is important for heart health.

C. Ginkgo biloba: Incorrect. Ginkgo biloba is used for its antioxidant properties and is commonly associated with improving memory. It does not have a significant impact on cholesterol levels.

D. Chamomile: Incorrect. Chamomile has antispasmodic and anti-inflammatory effects and produces a mild sedative effect. It is used primarily for digestive issues and relaxation rather than for managing cholesterol levels or cardiovascular health.

Administration of Blood Products

Which of the following is a common symptom of circulatory overload during a blood transfusion?

A) Sudden chills and high fever

B) Cough and shortness of breath

C) Red-colored urine

D) Twitchy reflexes and muscle cramps

Correct Answer: B) Cough and shortness of breath

Explanation:

A) Sudden chills and high fever: This is a sign of septicemia, not circulatory overload.

B) Cough and shortness of breath: These are hallmark symptoms of circulatory overload.

C) Red-colored urine: This is associated with iron overload treatment, not circulatory overload.

D) Twitchy reflexes and muscle cramps: These are signs of hypocalcemia.

Que: What is the immediate action when circulatory overload is suspected during a blood transfusion?

A) Increase the infusion rate

B) Stop the infusion and position the patient flat

C) Slow the infusion and adjust the patient's position

D) Administer antibiotics

Correct Answer: C) Slow the infusion and adjust the patient's position

Explanation:

A) Increase the infusion rate: This would worsen circulatory overload, making the situation more critical.

B) Stop the infusion and position the patient flat: The correct position is sitting upright with legs lowered, not flat.

C) Slow the infusion and adjust the patient's position: This is the proper initial response when circulatory overload is suspected.

D) Administer antibiotics: This action is appropriate for septicemia, not circulatory overload.

Which of the following conditions is most commonly associated with citrate toxicity during blood transfusions?

A) Rapid infusion of multiple blood units

B) Presence of blood microorganisms

C) Multiple transfusions leading to excess iron

D) Blood transfusion from an unscreened donor

Correct Answer: A) Rapid infusion of multiple blood units

Explanation:

A) Rapid infusion of multiple blood units: This is the main cause of citrate toxicity, especially in patients with liver issues.

B) Presence of blood microorganisms: This refers to septicemia, not citrate toxicity.

C) Multiple transfusions leading to excess iron: This describes iron overload, not citrate toxicity.

D) Blood transfusion from an unscreened donor: This increases the risk of disease transmission, not citrate toxicity.

Que: Which electrolyte imbalance is most likely to result from the release of potassium from stored blood during a transfusion?

A) Hypocalcemia

B) Hyperkalemia

C) Citrate toxicity

D) Septicemia

Correct Answer: B) Hyperkalemia

Explanation:

A) Hypocalcemia: This occurs due to citrate binding to calcium, not potassium release.

B) Hyperkalemia: Potassium release from stored blood leads to hyperkalemia.

C) Citrate toxicity: This is related to citrate accumulation, not potassium release.

D) Septicemia: This results from microorganisms in transfused blood, not electrolyte imbalances.

Que : Which of the following is a primary preventive measure to avoid disease transmission during blood transfusions?

A) Administering deferoxamine

B) Collecting blood cultures

C) Rigorous donor screening

D) Monitoring calcium levels

Correct Answer: C) Rigorous donor screening

Explanation:

A) Administering deferoxamine: This is a treatment for iron overload, not for disease transmission.

B) Collecting blood cultures: This is done when septicemia is suspected, not as a preventive measure.

C) Rigorous donor screening: This is the primary method for reducing disease transmission risks.

D) Monitoring calcium levels: This helps prevent hypocalcemia but does not prevent disease transmission.

Which solution type would be most appropriate for treating cellular dehydration without affecting extracellular fluid volume?

A) Hypertonic solutions

B) Isotonic solutions

C) Hypotonic solutions

D) Colloids

Correct Answer: C) Hypotonic solutions

Explanation:

A) Hypertonic solutions: Incorrect. Hypertonic solutions draw water out of cells into the extracellular space, which could worsen cellular dehydration.

B) Isotonic solutions: Incorrect. Isotonic solutions maintain fluid balance but do not specifically address cellular dehydration.

C) Hypotonic solutions: Correct. Hypotonic solutions help treat cellular dehydration by moving water into the cells, addressing cellular fluid deficits without significantly altering extracellular fluid volume.

D) Colloids: Incorrect. Colloids are used for expanding blood volume and are not specifically used for addressing cellular dehydration.

Managing Anaphylactic reactions

Practice Session

Que : Mrs. Agrima is a 55 year old woman with a history of severe allergies. She is currently being treated with a new medication for her allergies, but has experienced an anaphylactic reaction after taking the medication. Mrs. Agrima 's vital signs show a rapid, weak pulse and she is experiencing difficulty breathing. She has a skin rash and is nauseated and vomiting.

What should be the first action taken to manage Mrs. Agrima 's anaphylactic reaction?

A) Administer epinephrine or adrenaline

B) Stop the medication that is causing the reaction

C) Elevate the head of the bed

D) Check the ABCs (Airway, Breathing, and Circulation)

The first action to manage Mrs. Agrima's anaphylactic reaction should be:

A) Administer epinephrine or adrenaline

Explanation:

Administering epinephrine is the first-line treatment for anaphylaxis. It works quickly to reverse the symptoms by constricting blood vessels, improving blood pressure, relaxing the muscles in the airways, and reducing swelling and hives.

Other Options:

B) Administer oxygen

Explanation: Administering oxygen is important to support breathing, but it is not the immediate first action. Epinephrine is needed to quickly counteract the severe allergic reaction.

C) Elevate the head of the bed

Explanation: Elevating the head of the bed can help with breathing, but it is not the first action. The immediate administration of epinephrine is crucial.

D) Check the ABCs (Airway, Breathing, and Circulation)

Explanation: Checking the ABCs is important in any emergency situation, but in the case of anaphylaxis, administering epinephrine takes precedence to quickly reverse the severe allergic reaction.

> **Managing an anaphylactic reaction requires prompt and decisive action to ensure the patient's safety and well-being. In the case of patient, who has experienced a severe allergic reaction to a medication, the first action should involve stopping the medication causing the reaction and checking the ABCs (Airway, Breathing, and Circulation). It is essential to ensure that the patient's airway is clear and they can breathe properly. Administering epinephrine or adrenaline is also crucial as it helps constrict blood vessels and open up airways, improving circulation and breathing. These measures, alongside monitoring vital signs and providing supportive care such as fluids, form the cornerstone of managing an anaphylactic reaction. Additionally, identifying and avoiding triggers for future reactions and educating the patient about their allergies are vital components of long-term management. Swift and appropriate intervention can significantly improve outcomes for patients experiencing anaphylaxis.**

Disaster Planning

tip **FEMA categorizes disasters into three levels: Level 1 involves full federal involvement, Level 2 entails moderate federal support, and Level 3 indicates minor disasters with limited federal aid. Nurses, vital members of disaster response teams, participate in preparedness activities like emergency drills and receive training in disaster management and CPR. Personal and professional readiness is crucial for nurses to fulfill their roles effectively while understanding their hospital's disaster management plan. Disaster management encompasses mitigation, preparedness, response, and recovery phases, with nurses playing key roles in each phase. They provide swift actions during the response phase, including triage and wound care, and contribute to recovery efforts by offering medical care, emotional support, and rehabilitation post-disaster. Collaboration and effective communication within nursing staff are facilitated through the creation of disaster response groups.**

Practice Session

Que: A wildfire breaks out in a national park, prompting the need for immediate action to save lives and contain the fire. There is no presidential emergency declaration at the initial stage. Which phase of disaster management does this situation primarily fall under, according to the information provided?

A) Mitigation

B) Preparedness

C) Response

D) Recovery

Answer: C) Response

Explanation: In the given scenario, a wildfire has broken out, and the immediate need is to take actions to save people's lives and contain the fire. This aligns with the definition of the "Response" phase in disaster management, which involves taking actions to save people's lives in the wake of a disaster. Option A) Mitigation involves actions taken to reduce the damage caused by a disaster, which is not the primary focus in this situation. Option B) Preparedness involves planning and being ready for a disaster, but the situation described is beyond the planning stage. Option D) Recovery involves restoring the situation to its condition prior to the disaster, which is not the immediate concern in this scenario.

Que : Match the following disaster situations to their appropriate FEMA disaster response levels.

Disaster Situations:

A local wildfire is managed entirely by local fire departments with no federal support.

A major hurricane strikes a coastal city, causing significant damage and requiring substantial federal assistance.

A severe drought impacts several states, prompting state and federal resources for relief efforts.

A localized tornado causes damage to a small town, and local authorities handle the situation without federal intervention.

FEMA Disaster Response Levels:

A. Level 1 Disaster

B. Level 2 Disaster

C. Level 3 Disaster

D. Level 4 Disaster

Matching:

A local wildfire is managed entirely by local fire departments with no federal support.

C. Level 3 Disaster

Explanation: This situation matches Level 3, where the disaster is managed entirely by local resources with no federal involvement.

A major hurricane strikes a coastal city, causing significant damage and requiring substantial federal assistance.

A. Level 1 Disaster

Explanation: This situation fits Level 1, where a major disaster requires full federal involvement and support.

A severe drought impacts several states, prompting state and federal resources for relief efforts.

B. Level 2 Disaster

Explanation: This describes Level 2, where there is significant state and federal involvement, but not as extensive as Level 1.

A localized tornado causes damage to a small town, and local authorities handle the situation without federal intervention.

C. Level 3 Disaster

Explanation: This situation is correctly identified as Level 3, where local authorities manage the disaster without federal assistance.

Note: Level 4 Disaster is not used in FEMA's classification system and is not applicable to the situations provided.

Prioritization

Before diving into a practice session, keep in mind these key prioritization strategies:

Carefully read the entire question, focusing on key phrases that hint at what is being asked.

Identify the client's priority needs, considering physiological, safety, psychological, and spiritual factors.

Narrow down your choices by identifying the correct nursing diagnosis for the client's issue.

Ensure the answer falls within the RN's scope of practice, avoiding actions reserved for advanced practitioners.

Assess the urgency of the situation, determining whether it requires immediate intervention.

Evaluate the potential risk for harm, selecting options that minimize risk to the client.

Consider the client's cultural or religious beliefs and how they might affect care decisions.

Prioritize options backed by current evidence-based practices.

Utilize critical thinking to balance all the information, weighing pros and cons before deciding.

Practice frequently to build confidence and improve your prioritization skills.

Additionally:

Maslow's Hierarchy of Needs is crucial for judging priorities—always address physiological needs first, followed by safety, social, esteem, and self-actualization.

Prioritization can be broken into high, intermediate, and low categories, with life-threatening conditions like airway management at the highest level (use ABC: Airway, Breathing, Circulation).

Non-life-threatening but timely interventions, such as monitoring vital signs, fall into intermediate priorities.

Low-priority actions, like preventing bedsores, come last but still matter.

Resource management and rational judgment, factoring in patient condition and available resources, are essential.

Effective communication with the patient, family, and team ensures proper prioritization.

Continuously reassess priorities as conditions evolve.

Experience and knowledge, gained through training and practice, enhance clinical judgment and prioritization skills.

Scenario:

Nurse Elena is caring for Mr. Johnson, a 60-year-old patient with multiple health issues. He has recently been admitted to the hospital with chest pain, shortness of breath, and a history of diabetes and hypertension. Upon assessment, Nurse Elena identifies several needs:

A. Immediate pain relief for severe chest pain.
B. Monitoring and managing blood glucose levels due to diabetes.
C. Providing patient education on hypertension management.
D. Discussing lifestyle changes for long-term health improvement.

Que :

Based on the prioritization guidelines, which of the following actions should Nurse Elena take first?

A) Educate Mr. Johnson about hypertension management.

B) Discuss lifestyle changes for long-term health improvement.

C) Manage and monitor Mr. Johnson's blood glucose levels.

D) Provide immediate pain relief for severe chest pain.

Correct Answer:

D) Provide immediate pain relief for severe chest pain.

Explanation:

A) Educate Mr. Johnson about hypertension management: This is incorrect as it is not the most urgent issue. Although patient education is important, it does not address the immediate and life-threatening concern of severe chest pain.

B) Discuss lifestyle changes for long-term health improvement: This is incorrect because discussing lifestyle changes is relevant for long-term management but does not address the immediate or urgent health needs.

C) Manage and monitor Mr. Johnson's blood glucose levels: This is a necessary intervention but is not as critical as addressing severe chest pain. Managing blood glucose is important for overall health but does not take priority over life-threatening issues.

D) Provide immediate pain relief for severe chest pain: This is correct. Severe chest pain is a potential sign of a life-threatening condition, such as a heart attack. According to the prioritization guidelines, addressing life-threatening issues, like severe chest pain, takes precedence over less urgent needs.

Que: Nurse Maria is caring for a patient who has difficulty breathing, complains of abdominal pain, and expresses concern about being away from her family during her hospital stay. Nurse Maria must decide which of these issues to address first.

Which of the following situations should Nurse Maria prioritize first when providing care?

A) The patient's concern about being away from her family

B) The patient's complaint of abdominal pain

C) The patient's difficulty breathing

D) The patient's request for help with personal hygiene

E) The patient's need for assistance with documentation for discharge

Correct Answer:

C) The patient's difficulty breathing

Explanation:

A (Incorrect): While the patient's emotional concerns are important, they do not take precedence over physical health issues, especially when there is a threat to life.

B (Incorrect): Abdominal pain can be distressing, but it is not immediately life-threatening. Breathing issues should be prioritized first.

C (Correct): Difficulty breathing is a life-threatening issue and should be addressed immediately according to the ABCs of emergency care, where airway takes priority.

D (Incorrect): Personal hygiene, while important for comfort, is a low-priority concern compared to breathing difficulties.

E (Incorrect): Documentation for discharge is not an urgent issue and can be addressed once the patient's immediate health concerns are resolved.

Nurse John is caring for a patient who has a low-grade fever, a history of heart disease, and is complaining of chest tightness. The patient also mentions feeling anxious about their upcoming surgery. Nurse John must determine which issue to address first.

Which of the following situations should Nurse John prioritize first when providing care?

A) The patient's anxiety about the upcoming surgery

B) The patient's complaint of chest tightness

C) The patient's low-grade fever

D) The patient's request for information about their medication

E) The patient's need for assistance with walking

Correct Answer:

B) The patient's complaint of chest tightness

Explanation:

A (Incorrect): While anxiety is important, it is not life-threatening, especially when compared to physical symptoms that could indicate serious health risks.

B (Correct): Chest tightness in a patient with a history of heart disease is a potentially life-threatening condition and must be prioritized, as it could signal a heart attack or other critical cardiac issues.

C (Incorrect): A low-grade fever, though concerning, is not as urgent as chest tightness in a heart patient.

D (Incorrect): Medication information is important for the patient's knowledge but does not require immediate action compared to chest tightness.

E (Incorrect): While assisting with mobility is necessary, chest pain takes clear priority given its potential severity.

Delegation

Accountability: The delegator remains responsible for task completion.

Right Person for the Task: Ensure the delegate has appropriate training and skills.

Clear Communication: Provide precise instructions and verify understanding.

Supervision: Monitor task progress and provide feedback.

RN Tasks: Administer IV meds, plan care, train, and delegate.

LPN Tasks: Administer oral/injectable meds, catheterization, dressing changes.

UAP Tasks: Assist with hygiene, exercise, and ambulation.

Scope of Practice: Delegate within staff's capabilities and education level.

Risk Management: Identify and address potential risks.

Confidentiality: Ensure HIPAA compliance for sensitive tasks.

Nurse Amanda is overseeing a busy surgical unit. She needs to delegate tasks to her team. She plans to have an unlicensed assistive personnel (UAP) help with patient care in the recovery room.

Que : Which task is most appropriate for Nurse Amanda to delegate to the UAP?

A) Administering intravenous medication to a post-surgical patient.

B) Assisting a patient with range-of-motion exercises.

C) Performing a sterile dressing change on a surgical wound.

D) Reviewing the post-operative teaching plan with the patient.

Correct Answer: B) Assisting a patient with range-of-motion exercises.

Explanation:

- A) Administering intravenous medication to a post-surgical patient: This task requires the skills and qualifications of a registered nurse (RN) and cannot be delegated to a UAP.
- B) Assisting a patient with range-of-motion exercises: Correct. This is a noninvasive task that is appropriate for delegation to a UAP.
- C) Performing a sterile dressing change on a surgical wound: This task requires the expertise of an LPN or RN, as it involves invasive procedures.

- D) Reviewing the post-operative teaching plan with the patient: This task is the responsibility of an RN, who must assess and plan care, including patient education.

Scenario: Nurse Sarah is working in a long-term care facility and needs to delegate a task to an unlicensed assistive personnel (UAP). She needs to choose an appropriate task for the UAP.

Que : Which task is best suited for delegation to the UAP?

A) Monitoring a patient's blood glucose levels and interpreting results.

B) Performing a medication reconciliation with the patient.

C) Assisting a patient with eating and drinking during meals.

D) Teaching a patient how to manage their newly diagnosed hypertension.

Correct Answer: C) Assisting a patient with eating and drinking during meals.

Explanation:

- A) Monitoring a patient's blood glucose levels and interpreting results: This requires clinical skills and is typically performed by an LPN or RN.
- B) Performing a medication reconciliation with the patient: Medication reconciliation is a task for an RN, who is responsible for comprehensive patient assessments.
- C) Assisting a patient with eating and drinking during meals: Correct. This noninvasive, supportive task is suitable for a UAP.
- D) Teaching a patient how to manage their newly diagnosed hypertension: Patient education is a responsibility for an RN, who provides detailed information and guidance on health management.

Emergency Department Triage

In emergency department triage, the situation is prioritized based on the urgency of care required for patients.

The patients are classified into three groups: highest priority clients, urgent priority clients, and non-urgent clients.

The highest priority clients are those who have chances of survival with nursing intervention and need immediate attention. These patients require the highest caring priority.

Examples of such cases are acute heart conditions, stroke, clients with amputated limbs, acute chemical effects on eyes, acute respiratory attacks, chest pain, burns, and hypersensitive reactions.

Urgent priority clients or intermediate priority clients are those who have non-life threatening injuries. These patients require medical service within 30 minutes to 120 minutes.

Examples of such cases are patients with open fractures, wounds, and medium burns.

Non-urgent clients or least priority clients are those who do not have life-threatening complications and can wait for 2 hours for a healthcare worker.

Examples of such cases are muscle strain, ligament strain, and closed fracture.

Practice Session

A 45-year-old man arrives at the emergency department following a car accident. He is unconscious, has severe chest pain, and is showing signs of respiratory distress. The attending nurse needs to classify his triage priority.

Que : Which triage priority should be assigned to this patient?

A) Urgent (Yellow)

B) Nonurgent (Green)

C) Emergent (Red)

D) Black

Correct Answer:

C) Emergent (Red)

Explanation:

A) Urgent (Yellow): Incorrect. This classification is for patients needing treatment within 30 minutes to 2 hours, not for those with life-threatening conditions.

B) Nonurgent (Green): Incorrect. This classification is for patients with minor injuries who can wait for treatment for at least 2 hours.

C) Emergent (Red): Correct. The patient has life-threatening injuries and requires immediate attention. His severe chest pain and respiratory distress indicate a high probability of survival if stabilized.

D) Black: Incorrect. The patient is not dead or likely to die imminently; he requires urgent care.

In the emergency department, a nurse is assigned to prioritize patients based on their conditions. Below are the statements from the nurse about five different patients:

1. **Patient A**: "This patient has severe chest pain and difficulty breathing, which started about an hour ago."
2. **Patient B**: "This patient sustained a moderate burn on their forearm. They are stable and in moderate pain."
3. **Patient C**: "This patient has a sprained ankle and can walk with minimal assistance. There is no sign of a fracture."
4. **Patient D**: "This patient has a wound that is actively bleeding but not severely. The bleeding has been managed with a pressure bandage."
5. **Patient E**: "This patient has suddenly lost movement in their right arm and is experiencing slurred speech, which started 20 minutes ago."

Multiple Choice Question

Which of the following patients should be given the highest priority for care in the emergency department? (Select TWO correct answers)

- A. Patient A
- B. Patient B
- C. Patient C
- D. Patient D
- E. Patient E

Explanation of Options:

1. **Option A (Patient A: Severe chest pain and difficulty breathing) - Correct**
    - **Reasoning**: Patient A is experiencing symptoms that may indicate a life-threatening condition, such as a heart attack or respiratory failure. Chest pain and difficulty breathing

are red flags for acute cardiovascular or respiratory events, which require immediate medical intervention. This makes Patient A a **highest priority client**.

2. **Option B (Patient B: Moderate burn on forearm) - Incorrect**
   - **Reasoning**: Patient B has a moderate burn, which is a non-life-threatening injury. This patient falls under the **urgent priority client** category and requires attention within 30 to 120 minutes but not immediate care. Therefore, they are not the highest priority.

3. **Option C (Patient C: Sprained ankle, no fracture) - Incorrect**
   - **Reasoning**: Patient C has a sprained ankle without a fracture and can walk with assistance, indicating that the condition is stable and non-life-threatening. This makes Patient C a **non-urgent client**, meaning they can wait for more than 2 hours for medical attention. Thus, they do not need immediate intervention.

4. **Option D (Patient D: Wound with managed bleeding) - Incorrect**
   - **Reasoning**: Patient D has a wound with managed bleeding, and although it requires medical evaluation, the bleeding is controlled. This situation falls under the **urgent priority client** category as the condition is not life-threatening. This patient does not need immediate care compared to others with potentially life-threatening conditions.

5. **Option E (Patient E: Sudden loss of movement and slurred speech) - Correct**
   - **Reasoning**: Patient E is showing symptoms consistent with a possible stroke, such as sudden loss of movement and slurred speech. A stroke requires immediate intervention to prevent further brain damage and to improve chances of recovery. This makes Patient E a **highest priority client**.

Correct Answers: A and E. Both patients are experiencing symptoms that may indicate life-threatening conditions and require immediate medical intervention.

ACID BASE BALANCE

- A nurse needs to know the acid-base balance of a patient for which ABG test can be helpful.
- ABG test involves measuring pH, PaCO2, HCO3, oxygen saturation (O2 Sat), and PaO2.
- pH determines if it is an acidotic or alkalotic condition.
- PaCO2 measures carbon dioxide in blood, which indicates respiratory acidosis or alkalosis.
- HCO3 acts as a buffer in maintaining pH.
- O2 Sat measures the percentage of oxygen bound to hemoglobin, and the normal range is 94-100%.
- PaO2 shows the combining capacity of oxygen with hemoglobin, and the normal range is 80-100 mmHg.
- Oxygen content and oxygen saturation are different concepts.
- Normal ranges for ABG parameters are: pH (7.35-7.45), PaCO2 (35-45 mmHg), HCO3 (22-26 mEq/L), O2 Sat (94-100%), and PaO2 (80-100 mmHg).

- Metabolic acidosis: Decreased pH, pCO2, and decreased bicarbonate
- Metabolic alkalosis: Elevated pH, pCO2, and bicarbonate
- Respiratory acidosis: Decreased pH and elevated pCO2 and bicarbonate
- Respiratory alkalosis: Elevated pH and decreased pCO2 and bicarbonate

Respiratory Acidosis:
- Caused by excess hydrogen ion in blood when buffer system is insufficient.
- Hypoventilation is a major cause.
- Conditions causing respiratory obstruction or airway inflammation can cause respiratory acidosis.
- Clinical manifestations include hypoventilation, increased urine acid levels, drowsiness, seizures, dysrhythmia, headache, and coma.
- Nursing interventions include suctioning, administration of oxygen, deep breathing, and coughing. Do not prescribe opioids or respiratory depressants to treat restlessness.

Respiratory Alkalosis:
- Caused by hyperventilation of the lungs.
- Conditions causing overstimulation of the respiratory system can cause respiratory alkalosis.
- Symptoms include neuromuscular symptoms, tachycardia, dysrhythmia, lethargy, confusion, nausea, vomiting, and pain.
- Nursing interventions include calming the patient, using the rebreathing technique, administering calcium gluconate, teaching relaxation techniques, and prescribing opioids.

Metabolic Acidosis:
- Occurs when there is increased acid or loss of bicarbonates in the body
- Causes include kidney disease, diarrhea, and lactic acidosis
- Symptoms include hyperventilation, fatigue, confusion, and cardiac arrhythmias
- Nursing interventions include treating the underlying cause, administering bicarbonate, and monitoring electrolyte levels

Metabolic Alkalosis:
- Occurs when there is a significant loss of acid or increase in bicarbonates in the body
- Causes include excessive vomiting or use of diuretics
- Symptoms include confusion, twitching, and muscle weakness
- Nursing interventions include treating the underlying cause, administering chloride or ammonium, and monitoring electrolyte levels.

NGN Case Study

Patient Profile:

Name: Nikita S.

Age: 45

Medical History: Nikita S. has a history of chronic obstructive pulmonary disease (COPD) and has been a heavy smoker for the past 20 years.

Presenting Complaint: Nikita S. is admitted to the emergency department with complaints of severe shortness of breath, confusion, and muscle weakness. She also mentions that she has been experiencing excessive vomiting for the past 24 hours.

Case Scenario: Upon examination, Nikita S.'s vital signs are as follows:

Blood pressure: 150/90 mm Hg

Heart rate: 110 beats per minute

Respiratory rate: 30 breaths per minute

Oxygen saturation: 88% on room air

Laboratory Results:

Arterial blood gas analysis: pH of 7.48 (alkaline)

PaCO2 (partial pressure of carbon dioxide): 28 mm Hg (lower than normal)

HCO3- (bicarbonate) level: 32 mEq/L (higher than normal)

Potassium (K+) level: 2.9 mEq/L (lower than normal)

Que : Which acid-base imbalance is Nikita S. most likely experiencing, and what are the possible causes?

A) Respiratory Acidosis due to COPD

B) Respiratory Alkalosis due to hyperventilation

C) Metabolic Acidosis due to kidney disease

D) Metabolic Alkalosis due to excessive vomiting

E) Respiratory Acidosis due to hyperventilation

F) Metabolic Alkalosis due to diuretic use

G) Respiratory Alkalosis due to diarrhea

Correct Answer: D) Metabolic Alkalosis due to excessive vomiting

Explanation:

Metabolic Alkalosis (Option D) is indicated by an alkaline pH (above 7.45) and an elevated bicarbonate (HCO3-) level. In Nikita S.'s case, her pH is alkaline (7.48), and her bicarbonate level is higher than normal (32 mEq/L). Excessive vomiting can lead to the loss of gastric acid, resulting in metabolic alkalosis.

Respiratory Compensation: The low PaCO2 (28 mm Hg) indicates respiratory compensation for the metabolic alkalosis. The body tries to compensate for the alkalosis by reducing CO2 levels through hyperventilation.

The other options (A, B, C, E, F, G) do not align with Nikita S.'s clinical presentation and laboratory results:

> Option A (Respiratory Acidosis due to COPD) is not supported by her low PaCO2 level.
>
> Option B (Respiratory Alkalosis due to hyperventilation) is not consistent with her clinical scenario of vomiting.
>
> Option C (Metabolic Acidosis due to kidney disease) is not consistent with her alkaline pH.
>
> Option E (Respiratory Acidosis due to hyperventilation) contradicts her alkaline pH.
>
> Option F (Metabolic Alkalosis due to diuretic use) is not relevant as there is no mention of diuretic use.
>
> Option G (Respiratory Alkalosis due to diarrhea) does not account for her symptoms of excessive vomiting.

In summary, Nikita S. is experiencing metabolic alkalosis due to the loss of gastric acid resulting from her vomiting.

Acid-base balance, monitored through ABG (Arterial Blood Gas) tests, is crucial for patient health. The test measures pH, PaCO2, HCO3, O2 Sat, and PaO2 to assess acidosis or alkalosis. Respiratory acidosis, alkalosis, metabolic acidosis, and alkalosis manifest differently and require specific nursing interventions. For instance, addressing excess hydrogen ions and providing oxygen for respiratory acidosis, or treating underlying causes like kidney disease for metabolic acidosis. Nurses play a vital role in interpreting ABG results and implementing interventions to restore balance and ensure patient well-being.

Case Study

Patient Profile:
- **Name:** Kurrim

- **Age:** 45
- **Gender:** Male
- **Medical History:** Kurrim was admitted to the hospital with complaints of shortness of breath and confusion.

    Scenario: Kurrim's medical team suspects an acid-base imbalance. To assess his condition, the nurse orders an Arterial Blood Gas (ABG) test. The ABG results are as follows:

- **pH:** 7.25 (Below the normal range)
- **PaCO2:** 50 mmHg (Above the normal range)
- **HCO3:** 24 mEq/L (Within the normal range)
- **O2 Sat:** 92% (Within the normal range)
- **PaO2:** 75 mmHg (Within the normal range)

    Que : What is the primary acid-base disturbance indicated by Kurrim's ABG results?

    A) Metabolic Acidosis

    B) Metabolic Alkalosis

    C) Respiratory Acidosis

    D) Respiratory Alkalosis

    Answer: C) Respiratory Acidosis

    Explanation: To determine the primary acid-base disturbance, let's analyze the ABG results:

- **pH** is below the normal range (7.25), indicating acidosis.
- **PaCO2** is above the normal range (50 mmHg), suggesting respiratory acidosis.
- **HCO3** is within the normal range (24 mEq/L), which does not indicate a primary metabolic disturbance.

    Based on these findings, it is apparent that there is an acidosis, and the elevated PaCO2 points toward respiratory acidosis as the primary disturbance. Therefore, option C, Respiratory Acidosis, is the correct answer.

    Now, let's briefly explain why the other options are incorrect:

- **Option A (Metabolic Acidosis):** This is not the correct answer because the primary disturbance is related to elevated PaCO2, not a metabolic issue.
- **Option B (Metabolic Alkalosis):** This is not the correct answer because the pH is below the normal range, indicating acidosis.
- **Option D (Respiratory Alkalosis):** This is not the correct answer because the pH is below the normal range, indicating acidosis.

    In summary, the ABG results point to **respiratory acidosis** as the primary acid-base disturbance in this case.

Electrolytes

ION Normal Serum Concentration In mEq/L or mg/dL

Sodium: 135 to 145 mEq/L
Potassium: 3.5 to 5.0 mEq/L
Calcium: 9 to 10.5 mg/dL
Magnesium: 1.3 to 2.1 mEq/L
Phosphorus: 3 to 4.5 mg/dL

- Hypokalemia: ST depression with inverted and flat T waves, watch for prominent U wave.
- Hyperkalemia: Tall T waves, flat P waves, Widened PR and QRS intervals.
- Hypocalcemia: Wide ST and QT intervals.
- Hypercalcemia: Short ST interval with wide T waves.
- Hypomagnesemia: Depressed ST with tall T waves.
- Hypermagnesemia: Wide QRS and PR intervals.
- Potassium Administration: It is crucial not to administer potassium intramuscularly, through IV push, or subcutaneously due to the potential for tissue damage.

Que: Which of the following electrocardiographic changes is associated with hypocalcemia?

A) Shortened ST segment and widened T wave

B) Prolonged QT interval and prolonged ST segment

C) ST depression and prominent U waves

D) Prolonged PR interval and flattened T wave

E) Shortened QT interval and flattened ST segment

Correct Answer:

B) Prolonged QT interval and prolonged ST segment

Rationale:

A) Shortened ST segment and widened T wave: This is indicative of hypercalcemia, not hypocalcemia. Hypercalcemia typically results in a shortened ST segment and a widened T wave.

B) Prolonged QT interval and prolonged ST segment: This is correct for hypocalcemia. Hypocalcemia causes a prolonged QT interval and ST segment on an ECG.

C) ST depression and prominent U waves: These changes are associated with hypokalemia, not hypocalcemia.

D) Prolonged PR interval and flattened T wave: These are not characteristic of hypocalcemia. Prolonged PR interval and flattened T wave can be seen with other conditions but are not specifically linked to hypocalcemia.

E) Shortened QT interval and flattened ST segment: This pattern is associated with hypercalcemia, not hypocalcemia. Hypocalcemia is characterized by a prolonged QT interval and ST segment.

NGN Case Study

Patient's History: Mr. Saigrace, a 65-year-old male, was admitted to the hospital with complaints of confusion, muscle weakness, and seizures. His past medical history was significant for high blood pressure and diabetes. He was on diuretic medications for the past few months. On examination, his blood pressure was found to be low and his pulse was weak.

Nurse's Notes: 1/31, Admitted with complaints of confusion, muscle weakness, and seizures.

BP: 90/60 mmHg, Pulse: weak PMH: HTN, DM On diuretic meds 2/1, Sodium level: 125 mEq/L (Hyponatremia) Started on sodium chloride IV infusions. Potassium level: 3.2 mEq/L (Hypokalemia)

Physician's Order:

- Sodium chloride IV infusion
- Monitor electrolyte levels
- Reduce dose of diuretic medication
- Dietary restriction of sodium

Lab Values: Sodium: 125 mEq/L Potassium: 3.2 mEq/L

Que A. What is the most likely cause of the patient's confusion, muscle weakness, and seizures?

A) Hypertension

B) Diabetes Mellitus

C) Hyponatremia

D) Hypokalemia

E) Diuretic medication

Correct Options: C) Hyponatremia and D) Hypokalemia

Explanation:

- Hyponatremia (low sodium levels) is noted in the patient's lab values (125 mEq/L). Symptoms of hyponatremia include confusion, muscle weakness, and seizures, which are also present in the patient.

- Hypokalemia (low potassium levels) is also noted in the patient's lab values (3.2 mEq/L) and can cause similar symptoms.
- HTN and DM are present in the patient's PMH (past medical history), but are not the immediate cause of the symptoms.
- The diuretic medication the patient was on may have contributed to the low electrolyte levels, which is why the physician ordered to reduce the dose of the medication and monitor electrolyte levels. However, the main cause is the low sodium and potassium levels.

Que B. What is the most likely cause of the patient's hyponatremia and hypokalemia?

A. Excessive fluid intake

B. Increased use of diuretics

C. Kidney disease

D. Medication side effect

Answer: B. Increased use of diuretics

Explanation:

- The patient is admitted with symptoms of confusion, muscle weakness, and seizures and has a low blood pressure and weak pulse.
- The patient has a history of hypertension and diabetes and is on diuretic medication.
- The sodium level is low (125 mEq/L) and the potassium level is also low (3.2 mEq/L).
- The physician has ordered a reduction in the dose of diuretic medication and a dietary restriction of sodium.

These factors suggest that the increased use of diuretics is the most likely cause of the patient's hyponatremia and hypokalemia. Option A (excessive fluid intake) is not likely since the patient has a low blood pressure and is being monitored for electrolyte levels. Option C (kidney disease) may also contribute, but the focus is on reducing the dose of diuretics and dietary restrictions of sodium. Option D (medication side effect) is also a possibility, but the focus is on the patient's use of diuretics.

Que C. What is the correct nursing intervention for the patient with hyponatremia and hypokalemia as noted in the scenario?

A) Stop sodium chloride IV infusion

B) Increase dose of diuretic medication

C) No dietary restriction of sodium

D) Monitor fluid intake and output

Correct Option: D) Monitor fluid intake and output

Explanation: A) Stopping the sodium chloride IV infusion would be detrimental to the patient as they are suffering from hyponatremia, which is a low level of sodium in the blood. Sodium chloride infusion is necessary to replenish the sodium levels.

B) Increasing the dose of diuretic medication would further lower the potassium levels, as diuretics increase urine output and can result in the loss of potassium and other electrolytes.

C) No dietary restriction of sodium would not be appropriate as the patient is already suffering from hyponatremia, which could be due to excessive sodium intake. The dietary restriction of sodium is necessary to regulate sodium levels.

D) Monitoring fluid intake and output is important to ensure that the patient is not retaining excess fluid and electrolytes. This will help to regulate the electrolyte levels and prevent further fluctuations.

Que D. What nursing intervention should be taken for the patient's electrolyte imbalances?

A. Increase the dose of diuretic medication

B. Stop sodium chloride IV infusions

C. Remove dietary restriction of sodium

D. Monitor electrolyte levels

Correct Answer: D. Monitor electrolyte levels

Explanation: The physician has already ordered the appropriate interventions for the patient's electrolyte imbalances including sodium chloride IV infusion, reducing the dose of diuretic medication, and dietary restriction of sodium. The most important intervention at this point is to monitor the patient's electrolyte levels to ensure they are improving and within normal range.

Option A is incorrect because increasing the dose of diuretic medication may worsen the patient's hyponatremia and hypokalemia.

Option B is incorrect because stopping the sodium chloride IV infusions may result in further decline of the patient's sodium levels.

Option C is incorrect because removing the dietary restriction of sodium may lead to further imbalances in the patient's electrolyte levels.

Que E. What is the nursing intervention for Hyponatremia?

A. Provide sodium chloride IV infusions

B. Provide osmotic diuretics

C. Choose hormone replacement procedure

D. Reduce the dose of diuretics

Correct option: A. Provide sodium chloride IV infusions

Explanation: If Hyponatremia is due to fluid or blood loss, vomiting or diarrhea, the nursing intervention would be to provide sodium chloride IV infusions. Option B is not correct as osmotic diuretics are used in case of excess fluid volume and not in case of Hyponatremia. Option C is incorrect as it is only applicable if the cause is Addison's disease. Option D is correct only if the cause of Hyponatremia is due to certain medications such as diuretics.

Que F. What is the nursing intervention for hypokalemia?

A) Provide sodium chloride IV infusions

B) Administer diuretics

C) Supplement dietary potassium sources

D) Reduce the dose of drugs causing hypokalemia

Correct Option: C) Supplement dietary potassium sources

Explanation: Option A) is incorrect as hypokalemia is not caused by fluid or blood loss and does not require sodium chloride IV infusions.

Option B) is incorrect as the use of diuretics may further deplete potassium levels.

Option D) is incorrect as reducing the dose of drugs causing hypokalemia may not be enough to treat the condition and may require additional interventions.

Option C) is correct as supplementing dietary potassium sources such as bananas, spinach, or other green leafy vegetables can help to raise potassium levels in cases of moderately low potassium levels. However, severe hypokalemic states may require supplemental potassium.

Which of the following statements regarding electrolyte imbalances and their management are correct? (Select all that apply.)
A) Potassium can be safely administered intramuscularly.

B) Assessing renal function is unnecessary when managing electrolyte imbalances.

C) Osmotic diuretics are the treatment of choice for hyperkalemia.

D) Monitoring EKG changes is essential in patients with electrolyte imbalances.

E) There is no relationship between calcium and phosphorus levels.

F) Chvostek's sign is associated with hypercalcemia.

G) Trousseau's sign is unrelated to electrolyte imbalances.

H) Patients with hypercalcemia are at risk of fractures during movement.
Correct Answers: D, G, H

Explanation:
- D) Monitoring EKG changes helps assess the type and severity of electrolyte imbalances.
- G) Trousseau's sign is a sign of hypocalcemia, not hypercalcemia.
- H) Patients with hypercalcemia are at risk of fractures due to calcium leaching from bones, making them more fragile.

IV Solutions

Various types of intravenous (IV) solutions offer tailored treatments for different clinical scenarios. Ringer's Lactate, an isotonic solution, is utilized to address extracellular fluid loss stemming from burn injuries, bleeding, pancreatic conditions, or dehydration due to diarrhea. Nursing considerations include vigilant monitoring of electrolyte levels and fluid balance. The isotonic 0.9% Saline Solution serves to treat extracellular fluid loss and low sodium or chloride ion levels, often occurring after blood transfusions or metabolic acid/base imbalances, necessitating close monitoring of fluid balance and electrolyte levels. Dextrose Solution (D5W), initially isotonic but eventually becoming hypertonic, is employed to augment plasma or extracellular fluid loss; however, it cannot be used in isolation due to its lack of electrolytes, prompting the need for additional solutions and electrolyte monitoring. Similarly, 5% Dextrose in 0.225% Saline initially offers isotonic properties, transitioning to hypertonic, and is primarily used for maintenance fluid, warranting careful fluid balance monitoring. Conversely, 5% Dextrose in 0.9% Normal Saline, a hypertonic solution, is indicated for metabolic alkalosis and low sodium and chloride levels in the blood, mandating monitoring of fluid balance and electrolyte levels. 5% Dextrose in 0.45% Saline serves as hypertonic maintenance fluid, necessitating fluid balance supervision. Lastly, 5% Dextrose in Ringer's Lactate Solution, a hypertonic option, addresses extracellular fluid loss, mirroring the uses of Ringer's Lactate while requiring similar electrolyte and fluid balance monitoring. Understanding the concentrations, uses, and nursing considerations of these IV solutions is fundamental for providing effective patient care in various clinical contexts.

Practice Session

What is the primary use of colloids in medical treatment?

A) Increase intracellular fluid

B) Increase extracellular fluid

C) Rapidly expand blood volume

D) Cause water to move into the cells

Correct Answer: C) Rapidly expand blood volume

Explanation:

A) Increase intracellular fluid: Incorrect. Colloids don't affect the fluid inside cells.

B) Increase extracellular fluid: Incorrect. Colloids act by pulling fluid into the bloodstream, not just the extracellular fluid.

C) Rapidly expand blood volume: Correct. Colloids, also known as plasma expanders, are used to increase vascular volume quickly, particularly in emergencies like hemorrhage or hypovolemia.

D) Cause water to move into the cells: Incorrect. Colloids pull water from interstitial spaces into the bloodstream, not into cells.

Which type of solution increases extracellular fluid volume without causing a shift of fluid into the cells?

A) Hypotonic solutions

B) Hypertonic solutions

C) Isotonic solutions

D) Colloids

Correct Answer: C) Isotonic solutions

Explanation:

A) Hypotonic solutions: Incorrect. These cause water to move into cells, leading to potential cellular swelling.

B) Hypertonic solutions: Incorrect. These pull water out of the cells, not just increase extracellular fluid volume.

C) Isotonic solutions: Correct. Isotonic solutions have the same osmolality as body fluids and only increase extracellular fluid without fluid shifts into or out of cells.

D) Colloids: Incorrect. Colloids pull fluid from interstitial spaces into the bloodstream, not necessarily increasing extracellular fluid directly.

Case Study 1

Scenario: A patient arrives in the emergency room with severe dehydration and a history of persistent diarrhea. The patient's blood tests show low sodium levels.

Options:

Option A: Administer 0.9% Saline.

Option B: Administer Ringer's Lactate Solution.

Option C: Administer 5% Dextrose in Water (D5W).

Option D: Administer 5% Dextrose in 0.9% Saline (5% D/NS).

Correct Option: Option B: Administer Ringer's Lactate Solution.

Explanation:

The best option would be Option A: Administer 0.9% Saline. Here's why:

Severe dehydration and persistent diarrhea often lead to significant fluid and electrolyte loss.

0.9% Saline (normal saline) is an isotonic solution that helps to restore both fluid and sodium levels effectively.

It is particularly useful in cases of hyponatremia (low sodium levels), as it helps to correct the sodium deficit without causing a rapid shift in fluid balance.

Options B, C, and D might not be as appropriate in this case:

Ringer's Lactate Solution is isotonic and is effective for treating fluid loss from diarrhea and dehydration. But also note Ringer's Lactate Solution contains additional electrolytes like potassium and calcium, which might not be necessary and could complicate the electrolyte balance. So, given the situation, the other options could be better.

5% Dextrose in Water (D5W) is hypotonic and could potentially worsen hyponatremia by diluting the sodium levels further.

5% Dextrose in 0.9% Saline (5% D/NS) is hypertonic and might be used in specific situations but is generally not the first choice for initial rehydration and sodium correction.

Case Study 4

Scenario: A patient needs fluid replacement for ongoing maintenance after initial resuscitation, with a focus on providing more water compared to sodium.

Options:

Option A: Administer 5% Dextrose in 0.225% Saline (5% D/1/4 NS).

Option B: Administer 5% Dextrose in Ringer's Lactate Solution.

Option C: Administer 0.9% Saline.

Option D: Administer 5% Dextrose in 0.9% Saline (5% D/NS).

Correct Option: Option A: Administer 5% Dextrose in 0.225% Saline (5% D/1/4 NS).

Explanation:

Option A: 5% Dextrose in 0.225% Saline starts isotonic and is good for maintenance hydration due to its higher water content relative to sodium.

Option B: 5% Dextrose in Ringer's Lactate Solution is more suitable for initial resuscitation rather than maintenance.

Option C: 0.9% Saline is isotonic and not typically used for maintenance fluid with higher water content.

Option D: 5% Dextrose in 0.9% Saline is hypertonic and may not be ideal for ongoing maintenance.

Catheters and Tubing

Nursing management tips for catheters and tubing include monitoring for signs of discomfort or changes in output, removing them promptly when no longer needed to prevent complications, and practicing proper hand hygiene during insertion to prevent infections. Proper insertion technique is crucial to prevent complications like infection or injury. Patient education on the purpose and care of catheters and tubing is also essential for promoting understanding and compliance, while infection prevention measures, including sterile techniques, should always be observed.

Nursing Strategies for Catheters and Tubing

- **Proper Insertion Technique:**
- Follow protocols to avoid complications like infection or injury.

Example: Check nasogastric tube placement before administering meds or nutrition.

Infection Prevention:

- Use sterile techniques and practice hand hygiene.

Example: Clean the perineal area with gloves and position the urinary catheter drainage bag below bladder level.

Monitoring for Complications:

- Watch for blockages or dislodgement, and observe for discomfort or changes in output.

Example: Monitor nasogastric tube patients for pain, gagging, or vomiting.

Patient Education:

- Educate patients and families on catheter care, risks, and hygiene.

Example: Teach urinary catheter patients about hygiene and fluid intake to avoid blockages or infections.

Removal and Discontinuation:

- Remove catheters as soon as they're no longer needed.

Example: Ensure gentle removal of a urinary catheter and monitor for post-removal complications.

Practice Session

Que : Mr. Miranda, a 67-year-old patient, has been admitted to the hospital for treatment of pneumonia. Due to difficulty swallowing, he has a nasogastric tube in place for medication administration. The healthcare provider has ordered the administration of a crushed medication via the nasogastric tube. The nurse prepares to administer the medication.

Fill in the blanks question:

Before instilling the medication, the nurse should check the _____ and _____ contents.

A) respiratory rate and oxygen saturation

B) tube placement and residual

C) blood pressure and heart rate

D) temperature and weight

Correct Answer: B

Explanation:

Option A: Checking the respiratory rate and oxygen saturation is important for monitoring the patient's respiratory status but is not related to administering medication via a nasogastric tube.

Option B: This is the correct answer. Before instilling the medication, the nurse should check the tube placement and residual contents to ensure that the medication is being administered to the correct location and to prevent complications such as aspiration.

Option C: Checking the blood pressure and heart rate is important for monitoring the patient's cardiovascular status but is not related to administering medication via a nasogastric tube.

Option D: Checking the temperature and weight is important for monitoring the patient's overall health status but is not related to administering medication via a nasogastric tube.

> **tip** Understanding the purposes of nasogastric tubes - administering medications, facilitating colonoscopies, and removing lung mucus - is vital. Nurses must verify tube placement and residual contents before medication administration to prevent aspiration. For urinary catheterization in females, washing the perineal area with soap and water using clean gloves is crucial for infection prevention. Placing clients in a dorsal recumbent position, using the dominant hand for insertion while spreading labia with the non-dominant hand, and inflating the balloon appropriately ensure patient comfort and safety.

Which tube is characterized by having an expandable balloon at its distal end that is filled with a heavy substance for positioning?

A) Decompression Tube

B) Inflatable Tube

C) Double-Lumen Tube for Gastric Suction

D) Single-Lumen Drainage Tube

Correct Answer: B) Inflatable Tube

Explanation:

Option A: Decompression Tube has a balloon but is used for pressure relief in the small intestine, not for positioning.

Option B: Inflatable Tube has a small balloon filled with a heavy substance for positioning, which matches the description.

Option C: Double-Lumen Tube for Gastric Suction has two channels but does not include a balloon for positioning.

Option D: Single-Lumen Drainage Tube does not have an expandable balloon or heavy substance for positioning.

Which statement accurately describes a sign of tracheal stenosis?

A) The patient experiences a reduction in coughing and easy expectoration of secretions.

B) Tracheal stenosis commonly develops after the cuff is inflated.

C) Difficulty breathing and talking is a common symptom of tracheal stenosis.

D) Tracheal stenosis is indicated by a wide tracheal lumen observed after tube removal.

Correct Answer: C) Difficulty breathing and talking is a common symptom of tracheal stenosis.

Explanation:

Option A: Reduced coughing and easy expectoration of secretions are not consistent with tracheal stenosis, which typically causes increased coughing and difficulty with secretions.

Option B: Tracheal stenosis usually occurs after the cuff is deflated or the tube is removed, not when the cuff is inflated.

Option C: Difficulty with breathing and talking are common symptoms of tracheal stenosis due to the narrowed tracheal lumen, making this the correct choice.

Option D: Tracheal stenosis involves a narrowed tracheal lumen, not a wide one, so this statement is incorrect.

Que: Which of the following nursing management approaches are essential for the proper use of catheters and tubing? (Select all that apply)
A) Using non-sterile techniques during insertion

B) Monitoring for signs of discomfort or changes in output

C) Removing catheters and tubing as soon as they are no longer needed

D) Skipping patient education on the purpose and care of catheters

E) Practicing proper hand hygiene during catheter insertion

F) Inserting a nasogastric tube through the lungs

G) Ensuring the drainage bag is positioned above the level of the bladder

H) Cleaning the perineal area with soap and water using clean gloves

Correct Answers: B) Monitoring for signs of discomfort or changes in output, C) Removing catheters and tubing as soon as they are no longer needed, E) Practicing proper hand hygiene during catheter insertion, H) Cleaning the perineal area with soap and water using clean gloves

Explanation:
A) Using non-sterile techniques during insertion is incorrect because it goes against infection prevention principles. Sterile techniques should be used during catheter insertion and care.
B) Monitoring for signs of discomfort or changes in output is correct. Nurses should observe patients for signs of complications, such as blockages or dislodgement, and take appropriate action.
C) Removing catheters and tubing as soon as they are no longer needed is correct. This helps prevent complications and promotes patient comfort.
D) Skipping patient education on the purpose and care of catheters is incorrect. Patient education is an essential aspect of nursing management to promote understanding and compliance.
E) Practicing proper hand hygiene during catheter insertion is correct. Hand hygiene is crucial to prevent infections when handling catheters and tubing.
F) Inserting a nasogastric tube through the lungs is incorrect. It should be inserted into the stomach, not

the lungs, to prevent complications.

G) Ensuring the drainage bag is positioned above the level of the bladder is incorrect. The drainage bag should be positioned below the level of the bladder to prevent backflow of urine.

H) Cleaning the perineal area with soap and water using clean gloves is correct when caring for a patient with a urinary catheter to prevent infection.

!tip **Nursing management tips for catheters and tubing include monitoring for signs of discomfort or changes in output, removing them promptly when no longer needed to prevent complications, and practicing proper hand hygiene during insertion to prevent infections. Proper insertion technique is crucial to prevent complications like infection or injury. Patient education on the purpose and care of catheters and tubing is also essential for promoting understanding and compliance, while infection prevention measures, including sterile techniques, should always be observed.**

Que : A nurse has been asked to perform the urinary catheterization procedure on a female patient. Which of the following nursing actions should the nurse follow?

A) Place the client in a supine position.

B) Wash the perineal area with soap and water using clean gloves.

C) Spread labia with non-dominant hand while inserting the catheter.

D) Inflate balloon fully per manufacturer's directions.

Correct answer: B) Wash the perineal area with soap and water using clean gloves.

Explanation:

When performing the urinary catheterization procedure, it is important to follow the proper steps to prevent infection and ensure patient comfort.

Option A is incorrect as female clients should be placed in a dorsal recumbent position (supine with knees flexed) while male clients should be placed in a supine position with thighs slightly abducted.

Option C is incorrect as the dominant hand should be used to insert the catheter while the non-dominant hand should be used to spread labia.

Option D is incorrect as the balloon should be inflated fully, but the manufacturer's directions should not be followed blindly; rather, the nurse should be familiar with the appropriate amount of fluid to use.

Option B is the correct answer, as washing the perineal area with soap and water using clean gloves is an important step in preventing infection during the procedure. This step should be performed before applying a sterile drape and lubricating the catheter, and after removing and discarding gloves, hand hygiene should be performed.

> **tip** Understanding the purposes of nasogastric tubes - administering medications, facilitating colonoscopies, and removing lung mucus - is vital. Nurses must verify tube placement and residual contents before medication administration to prevent aspiration. For urinary catheterization in females, washing the perineal area with soap and water using clean gloves is crucial for infection prevention. Placing clients in a dorsal recumbent position, using the dominant hand for insertion while spreading labia with the non-dominant hand, and inflating the balloon appropriately ensure patient comfort and safety.

Which tube features two channels, with one channel used for suction and the other for administering a flushing solution to remove harmful substances from the stomach?

A) Double-Lumen Tube for Gastric Suction

B) Feeding Tube with Maintenance Port

C) Gastric Suction and Irrigation Tube

D) Single-Lumen Drainage Tube

Correct Answer: C) Gastric Suction and Irrigation Tube

Explanation:

Option A: Double-Lumen Tube for Gastric Suction has a smaller channel within a larger one for regulating suction pressure but does not include a flushing solution channel.

Option B: Feeding Tube with Maintenance Port is used for feeding and has a port for maintenance but does not have separate channels for suction and flushing.

Option C: Gastric Suction and Irrigation Tube is specifically designed with one channel for suction and another for irrigation, making it the correct choice.

Option D: Single-Lumen Drainage Tube is used for draining fluids and gases but does not feature a separate channel for flushing.

Infection Control

NGN Case Study

Patient History and Nurse's Notes:

Mrs. Martha Subedi, a 55-year-old female, underwent abdominal surgery for appendicitis three days ago. She has a history of type 2 diabetes managed with oral hypoglycemic agents. Mrs. Rodriguez is currently admitted to the surgical unit for postoperative care.

Nurse's Notes:

Postoperative recovery has been progressing as expected, with controlled pain and stable vital signs.

Mrs. Rodriguez complains of mild incisional pain but denies any signs of infection such as increased redness, swelling, or discharge.

Regular glucose monitoring reveals well-controlled blood sugar levels.

The surgical wound appears clean and dry, with intact staples in place.

Medications:

a) Ceftriaxone (Rocephin):

Purpose: Prophylactic antibiotic to prevent surgical site infection.

Dosage: 1g IV every 24 hours.

Duration: 48 hours postoperatively.

b) Acetaminophen (Tylenol):

Purpose: Pain management.

Dosage: 650mg orally every 4-6 hours as needed.

Vital Signs:

Blood Pressure: 120/80 mmHg (Normal range: 90/60 to 120/80 mmHg)

Heart Rate: 80 bpm (Normal range: 60 to 100 bpm)

Respiratory Rate: 18 bpm (Normal range: 12 to 20 bpm)

Temperature: 98.6°F (Normal range: 97.8 to 99.1°F)

Oxygen Saturation: 98% (Normal range: 95% to 100%)

Lab Reports:

Lab Reports:

a) White Blood Cell (WBC) Count:

Within normal range (Normal range: 4,000 to 11,000 cells/mcL).

b) Blood Glucose Level:

Within target range for a patient with diabetes (Normal range: 70 to 130 mg/dL).

c) C-reactive Protein (CRP):

Normal range, indicating no significant inflammation (Normal range: 0 to 1 mg/dL).

Que : Which aspect of Mrs. Rodriguez's postoperative status indicates successful infection control?

A) Increased redness around the surgical wound.

B) Complaints of mild incisional pain.

C) Stable vital signs and well-controlled blood sugar levels.

D) Discharge from the surgical wound.

E) Presence of intact staples.

Ans :

Explanation:

A) Increased redness around the surgical wound (Incorrect):

Redness is a sign of inflammation, which could indicate infection. Mrs. Rodriguez denies signs of infection, and the wound appears clean and dry, making increased redness unlikely.

B) Complaints of mild incisional pain (Incorrect):

Mrs. Rodriguez complains of mild incisional pain. Pain alone is not a reliable indicator of infection in this case.

C) Stable vital signs and well-controlled blood sugar levels (Correct):

Stable vital signs (blood pressure, heart rate, respiratory rate, temperature, and oxygen saturation) and well-controlled blood sugar levels indicate a favorable postoperative recovery without signs of infection.

D) Discharge from the surgical wound (Incorrect):

Discharge is a sign of infection, and Mrs. Rodriguez denies any signs of infection. The wound appears clean and dry, making the presence of discharge unlikely.

E) Presence of intact staples (Incorrect):

While intact staples are a positive sign, they alone do not confirm infection control. The overall assessment, including vital signs and absence of signs of infection, is more indicative of successful infection control.

Que : Which of the following statements by the nurse needs correction in the management and care of Mrs. Rodriguez, a postoperative patient?

A) "Administering Ceftriaxone for 48 hours postoperatively helps prevent surgical site infection."

B) "Acetaminophen is prescribed every 2 hours for effective pain management."

C) "Monitoring Mrs. Rodriguez's blood pressure, heart rate, and respiratory rate every 4 hours is sufficient."

D) "Pain assessment should include asking about the location, intensity, and quality of pain."

E) "Regular glucose monitoring is essential to ensure well-controlled blood sugar levels."

F) "The presence of mild incisional pain is expected during the early postoperative period."

G) "Inspecting the surgical wound for signs of infection is part of routine nursing care."

H) "Administering Ceftriaxone beyond 48 hours postoperatively enhances its prophylactic effects."

Ans :

Explanation:

A) "Administering Ceftriaxone for 48 hours postoperatively helps prevent surgical site infection." (Correct):

This statement is correct. Prophylactic antibiotics, like Ceftriaxone, are often prescribed for a specific duration postoperatively to prevent surgical site infections.

B) "Acetaminophen is prescribed every 2 hours for effective pain management." (Incorrect):

Acetaminophen is usually prescribed every 4-6 hours, not every 2 hours. This statement needs correction to avoid potential medication errors.

C) "Monitoring Mrs. Rodriguez's blood pressure, heart rate, and respiratory rate every 4 hours is sufficient." (Incorrect):

Monitoring vital signs every 4 hours may not be frequent enough during the early postoperative period. Continuous or more frequent monitoring may be necessary for early detection of any complications.

D) "Pain assessment should include asking about the location, intensity, and quality of pain." (Correct):

This statement is correct. Comprehensive pain assessment includes gathering information about the location, intensity, and quality of pain.

E) "Regular glucose monitoring is essential to ensure well-controlled blood sugar levels." (Correct):

This statement is correct. Regular glucose monitoring is crucial for patients with diabetes to maintain well-controlled blood sugar levels.

F) "The presence of mild incisional pain is expected during the early postoperative period." (Correct):

This statement is correct. Mild incisional pain is common in the early postoperative period, and it aligns with the expected recovery process.

G) "Inspecting the surgical wound for signs of infection is part of routine nursing care." (Correct):

This statement is correct. Routine inspection of the surgical wound is essential for early detection of any signs of infection.

H) "Administering Ceftriaxone beyond 48 hours postoperatively enhances its prophylactic effects." (Incorrect):

Continuing prophylactic antibiotics beyond the recommended duration may not necessarily enhance their effects and may contribute to antibiotic resistance. This statement needs correction.

In summary, the correct answers are B ("Acetaminophen is prescribed every 2 hours for effective pain management.") and C ("Monitoring Mrs. Rodriguez's blood pressure, heart rate, and respiratory rate every 4 hours is sufficient."), as these statements require correction in the context of nursing management and care of postoperative patients.

Que : Mrs. Rodriguez's blood glucose level is within the target range for a patient with diabetes, ranging from ____ to ____ mg/dL. This indicates that her diabetes is _____ controlled.

Options:

A) 50 to 150; moderately

B) 70 to 130; well

C) 90 to 180; poorly

D) 60 to 120; adequately

Ans : Explanation:

A) 50 to 150; moderately (Incorrect):

The correct blood glucose range for a patient with diabetes is not 50 to 150 mg/dL. This option provides an incorrect range and suggests moderate control, which is not supported by the case study.

B) 70 to 130; well (Correct):

The target range for blood glucose levels in a patient with diabetes is generally 70 to 130 mg/dL. This option provides the correct range, and the term "well" indicates that her diabetes is well-controlled, aligning with the information in the case study.

C) 90 to 180; poorly (Incorrect):

The correct blood glucose range is not 90 to 180 mg/dL. This option provides an incorrect range, and the term "poorly" suggests poor control, which is not supported by the case study.

D) 60 to 120; adequately (Incorrect):

The correct blood glucose range is not 60 to 120 mg/dL. This option provides an incorrect range, and the term "adequately" does not accurately describe the well-controlled blood glucose levels mentioned in the case study.

Que : Mrs. Rodriguez is prescribed Ceftriaxone, a prophylactic antibiotic, for ____ hours postoperatively to prevent surgical site infection. This antibiotic is administered at a dosage of ____ IV every 24 hours.

Options:

A) 24; 500mg

B) 48; 1g

C) 72; 750mg

D) 36; 2g

Ans :

Explanation:

A) 24; 500mg (Incorrect):

This option provides an incorrect duration and dosage for the administration of Ceftriaxone. The correct duration mentioned in the case study is longer, and the correct dosage is higher.

B) 48; 1g (Correct):

The case study mentions that Ceftriaxone is prescribed for 48 hours postoperatively at a dosage of 1g IV every 24 hours. This option accurately reflects the information provided.

C) 72; 750mg (Incorrect):

This option provides an incorrect duration and dosage for the administration of Ceftriaxone. The correct duration mentioned in the case study is shorter, and the correct dosage is lower.

D) 36; 2g (Incorrect):

This option provides an incorrect duration and dosage for the administration of Ceftriaxone. The correct duration mentioned in the case study is longer, and the correct dosage is lower.

In summary, the correct answer is B ("48; 1g"), as it accurately represents the prescribed duration and dosage of Ceftriaxone for prophylactic purposes based on the information provided in the case study.

Que : Which vital sign is most crucial to monitor for a patient with type 2 diabetes during the postoperative period?

A) Blood Pressure

B) Heart Rate

C) Blood Glucose Levels

D) Temperature

Correct Answer: C) Blood Glucose Levels

Explanation:

Option A: Blood Pressure is important for assessing cardiovascular health, but it is less critical for managing diabetes-related complications during the postoperative period compared to blood glucose levels.

Option B: Heart Rate provides information about cardiovascular status and response to stress, but it does not specifically address the concerns associated with diabetes management in the postoperative period.

Option C: Blood Glucose Levels are crucial to monitor because fluctuations can impact healing, increase the risk of complications, and affect overall recovery. Diabetes can cause significant changes in glucose mtabolism post-surgery, making this the most important vital sign to monitor.

Option D: Temperature is important for detecting infections or inflammatory responses but does not directly relate to the management of diabetes during the postoperative period.

Que : Which intervention is most effective for infection control in postoperative patients like Mrs. Rodriguez?

A) Administering pain medication regularly

B) Keeping the surgical wound moist for faster healing

C) Using strict aseptic techniques during wound care

D) Encouraging early ambulation for improved blood circulation

Explanation:

A) Administering pain medication regularly (Incorrect):

While pain management is important for postoperative patients, it is not a direct intervention for infection control. Infection control focuses on preventing and managing infections, and pain medication does not address this aspect.

B) Keeping the surgical wound moist for faster healing (Incorrect):

Keeping the surgical wound moist may contribute to wound healing, but it does not directly address infection control. In fact, excessive moisture can potentially create a breeding ground for bacteria, highlighting the importance of proper wound care.

C) Using strict aseptic techniques during wound care (Correct):

Strict aseptic techniques during wound care, such as using sterile instruments and maintaining a sterile field, are essential for infection control. This helps prevent the introduction of pathogens into the surgical site and reduces the risk of postoperative infections.

D) Encouraging early ambulation for improved blood circulation (Incorrect):

Early ambulation is beneficial for various aspects of postoperative recovery, including blood circulation, but it is not a direct intervention for infection control. Infection control measures focus on preventing and minimizing the risk of infections in postoperative patients.

Theories of Growth and Development

> **tip** The Theories of Growth and Development offer profound insights into the progression of human understanding and behavior. Here's a glimpse into some of the prominent theorists and their models:

Piaget's Cognitive Development Theory

Theorist: Jean Piaget

Key Ideas: Children actively construct their understanding of reality through hands-on experiences and interactions within their environment.

Developmental Stages: Sensorimotor, Preoperational, Concrete Operational, Formal Operational

Moral Development

Theorist: Lawrence Kohlberg

Key Concepts: Individuals advance through distinct stages of moral reasoning, which are shaped by their cognitive abilities and ethical perspectives.

Stages: Pre-conventional, Conventional, Post-conventional

Psychosexual Development

Theorist: Sigmund Freud

Key Tenets: Children progress through stages where they confront and resolve conflicts between their innate biological urges and societal expectations.

Developmental Phases: Oral, Anal, Phallic, Latency, Genital

Erik Erikson's Psychosocial Development Model

Theorist: Erik Erikson

Core Concepts: Individuals encounter a series of psychosocial challenges across eight developmental stages, each characterized by a unique crisis that demands resolution.

Stages: Trust vs. Mistrust, Autonomy vs. Shame and Doubt, Initiative vs. Guilt, Industry vs. Inferiority, Identity vs. Role Confusion, Intimacy vs. Isolation, Generativity vs. Stagnation, Ego Integrity vs. Despair

Practice Session

Que : Which of the following statements from the parents indicates that they are assisting their infant in achieving Erikson's stages of development?

A) "We have enrolled our infant in various extracurricular activities."
B) "We have left our infant to sleep alone in a separate room."
C) "We make sure to hold our infant often and meet their needs for food and hygiene."
D) "We encourage our infant to be independent and do things on their own."

The right answer is C) "We make sure to hold our infant often and meet their needs for food and hygiene." This option shows that the parents are providing a nurturing and supportive environment for their infant, which is crucial in Erikson's first stage of development, Trust vs. Mistrust.

Option A) "We have enrolled our infant in various extracurricular activities." is incorrect because infants are too young for extracurricular activities and this does not relate to Erikson's stages of development.
Option B) "We have left our infant to sleep alone in a separate room." is incorrect because infants need to feel safe and secure, and leaving them alone in a separate room can create a sense of fear and mistrust.
Option D) "We encourage our infant to be independent and do things on their own." is incorrect because infants are not yet at a stage where they can be independent, and this does not address their need for nurturing and support.

Que : Sarah is a 6-year-old girl who has been having difficulty controlling her bowel movements. Her parents are concerned and take her to the pediatrician. After a physical examination and ruling out any medical issues, the pediatrician explains to Sarah's parents that this may be related to her development and suggests they consult with a child psychologist. The psychologist explains to Sarah's parents that this may be related to the anal stage of Freud's psychosexual stages of development.

Which of the following statements from the psychologist is accurate regarding the anal stage of Freud's psychosexual stages of development for Sarah?

A. Sarah experiences pleasurable and conflicting feelings associated with the genital organs.
B. Sarah is concerned with self-gratification and operates on the Pleasure Principle.
C. Sarah gains pleasure from the elimination of feces and from their retention.
D. The conflict of this stage is between society's demands and sensations of pleasure associated with the mouth.
E. During this stage, Sarah develops satisfying sexual and emotional relationships with members of the opposite sex.
F. The individual gains gratification from their own body during the genital stage.

Correct answers: C and F.

Explanation:
Option A is incorrect because the pleasure and conflict feelings are associated with the genital organs during the phallic stage, not the anal stage. Option B is incorrect because it describes the oral stage, not the anal stage. Option D is incorrect because the conflict of the anal stage is between society's demands and sensations of pleasure associated with the anus, not the mouth. Option E is incorrect because it describes the genital stage, which occurs after the latency stage. Option C is correct because during the anal stage, children gain pleasure from the elimination of feces and from their retention. Option F is correct because the genital stage is when individuals gain gratification from their own body and develop satisfying sexual and emotional relationships with members of the opposite sex.

Que : A 4-month-old baby girl is brought to the pediatrician for a routine checkup. The doctor observes that the baby is grasping and switching objects from one hand to the other. Which of the following statements from the parents indicates that the baby is developing normally?

A) "She doesn't seem to recognize us yet, even though we're her parents."
B) "She cries a lot, especially when we put her down to sleep."
C) "She hasn't rolled over yet, but she seems to be trying."
D) "She loves it when we play with her and smile at her."

Answer: D) "She loves it when we play with her and smile at her."

Explanation: At 4 to 5 months, infants should be grasping and switching objects from one hand to the other, as well as showing enjoyment of social interaction. Option A is incorrect because at this age, infants should recognize and respond to their parents. Option B is incorrect because although infants may cry frequently, crying when put down to sleep specifically is not a developmental milestone. Option C is incorrect because rolling over is a milestone for 4 to 5 months, not a requirement for normal development at 4 months. Option D is correct because enjoyment of social interaction is a milestone for 4 to 5 months, and playing and smiling with the baby is a good indicator that she is meeting this milestone.

Preoperative Care

Patient Education: Explain knee replacement surgery, recovery expectations.

Example: Inform patient about post-op physical therapy sessions.

Medication Review: Check for allergies and review blood-thinning meds.

Example: Ensure patient stops aspirin before surgery.

NPO Guidelines: Advise fasting to prevent aspiration.

Example: Instruct patient to stop eating after midnight.

Pre-operative Testing: Conduct chest X-ray before lung surgery.

Example: Ensure respiratory health before procedure.

Consent and Documentation: Obtain consent, document risks.

Example: Patient signs form detailing surgery risks.

Anesthesia Assessment: Evaluate airway before administering anesthesia.

Example: Assess patient's anesthesia tolerance.

Infection Prevention: Administer antibiotics before surgery.

Example: Prevent surgical site infections.

Pre-operative Hygiene: Instruct patient to shower with antimicrobial soap.

Example: Reduce bacteria on skin before surgery.

Patient Positioning: Ensure proper alignment to prevent pressure injuries.

Example: Position patient correctly during spinal surgery.

Emotional Support: Offer reassurance and address concerns.

Example: Support patient anxious about upcoming surgery.

Practice Session

Que: Ms. Patel, a 40-year-old woman, is scheduled for abdominal surgery to remove a benign tumor. During the pre-operative assessment, the nurse asks Ms. Patel about her current medications and medical history to identify any potential risks during surgery.

Which of the following statements from the patient indicates that they may be at an increased risk of bleeding during surgery?

A) "I take antibiotics daily for a chronic infection."

B) "I take a medication for my high blood pressure."

C) "I take aspirin daily to prevent heart attacks."

D) "I take antidepressants for my depression."

Answer: C

Explanation:

• Option C: The use of aspirin, also known as acetylsalicylic acid, can interfere with platelet function and increase the risk of bleeding during surgery. Aspirin is commonly used as a blood thinner to prevent heart attacks and strokes, but its anticoagulant properties can pose a risk during surgical procedures.

Options A, B, and D may have implications for Ms. Patel's surgical outcome, but they do not directly increase the risk of bleeding during surgery. Antidepressants, antibiotics, and medications for high blood pressure are commonly prescribed medications that are generally not associated with an increased risk of bleeding during surgical procedures.

Que: Ms. Johnson, a 45-year-old woman, is scheduled for elective surgery to repair a herniated disc in her lumbar spine. As part of the pre-operative process, the nurse is responsible for obtaining informed consent from Ms. Johnson before the surgery.

Which of the following procedures is correct regarding nurse's role in obtaining informed consent?

A. Surgeon explains surgery and answers of questions.

B. Minors may need parent/guardian to sign consent.

C. Older clients may need legal guardian to sign consent.

D. Psychiatric clients can refuse treatment until legally determined unable to decide.

E. No sedation before client signs consent.

F. Phone consent from legal guardian/POA acceptable with witness.

G. Nurse ensures client understands surgery before signing consent.

H. Nurse documents witnessed consent after client acknowledges understanding.

Correct answers: G, H

Explanation:

Answer G is correct because the nurse ensures that the client understands the surgery before signing the consent. The responsibility of ensuring comprehension and clarity lies with the nurse rather than the surgeon. The nurse should clarify any doubts or questions the patient may have regarding the procedure.

Answer H is correct because the nurse documents the witnessed consent after the client acknowledges understanding. This documentation is crucial for legal and medical purposes, ensuring that the client's consent is properly recorded in the medical records.

Answer A is incorrect because although the surgeon may explain the surgery and answer questions, it is ultimately the nurse's responsibility to ensure that the patient understands and consents to the procedure.

Answer B is incorrect because while minors may need parental or legal guardian consent, this statement is not directly related to the nurse's role in obtaining informed consent.

Answer C is incorrect because the statement about older clients needing a legal guardian to sign consent is not specifically related to the nurse's responsibilities in obtaining informed consent.

Answer D is incorrect because it pertains to the rights of psychiatric clients to refuse treatment and is not directly related to the process of obtaining informed consent.

Answer E is incorrect because sedation should not be administered before the client signs the consent form to ensure that the patient is fully aware and able to make informed decisions.

Answer F is partially correct because obtaining telephone consent from a legal guardian or power of attorney for healthcare is acceptable, but it requires another nurse as a witness to ensure the validity of the consent given over the telephone.

Que: Mrs. Smith, a 65-year-old woman, is scheduled for surgery to repair a hip fracture following a fall at home. During the pre-operative assessment, the nurse asks Mrs. Smith about her current medications and medical history to identify any potential risks during surgery.

Which of the following statements from the patient indicates that they may be at an increased risk of bleeding during surgery?

A) "I take antibiotics daily for a chronic infection."

B) "I take a medication for my high blood pressure."

C) "I take aspirin daily to prevent heart attacks."

D) "I take antidepressants for my depression."

E) "I take a diuretic for my edema."

F) "I take insulin for my diabetes."

G) "I take an herbal supplement for my anxiety."

H) "I take a medication for my irregular heartbeat."

I) "I take a medication for my epilepsy."

Answer: C, H, I and G

Explanation:

• Option C: The use of acetylsalicylic acid (Aspirin), clopidogrel, and nonsteroidal anti-inflammatory drugs can alter platelet aggregation and increase the risk of bleeding during surgery. Aspirin, in particular, inhibits platelet function and can prolong bleeding time, posing a risk during surgical procedures.

• Option H: Medications used to manage irregular heartbeats, such as antidysrhythmics, can affect cardiac function and conduction during anesthesia, potentially increasing the risk of bleeding during surgery. They may interfere with the body's ability to maintain hemostasis and respond to bleeding.

Option G: Some herbal supplements containing ginko, biloba and ginseng can also cause bleeding risk.

• Option I: Long-term use of certain anticonvulsants can interfere with the metabolism of anesthetic agents and may contribute to coagulation disorders, increasing the risk of bleeding during surgery.

The other options (A, B, D, E, F, and G) may have implications for the surgical procedure and anesthesia management, but they do not directly influence the risk of bleeding during surgery. Antibiotics, medications for high blood pressure, antidepressants, diuretics, insulin, and herbal supplements generally do not affect hemostasis or increase bleeding risk to the same extent as aspirin, antidysrhythmics, and anticonvulsants.

Burn and Management

 **Types of Burn injuries and Nursing Management:**

I. Types of Burn injuries:
A. Based on depth of burns:

Superficial thickness burns- involving only epidermis with tingling sensation.
Superficial partial-thickness burns- affecting the dermis area with edema causing reduced blood supply.
Deep partial thickness burns- red on the surface and white on deep areas with moderate edema.
Full thickness burns- no skin sensation with waxy white yellow colorish skin and entire dermis and epidermis destroyed.
Deep full thickness burns- blackish with total lack of sensation and reaches internal bones, muscles and tissues.
B. Based on surface area:

Rule of nines- body surface area divided into percentages.

- The front and back of the head and neck equal 9% of the body's surface area.
- The front and back of each arm and hand equal 9% of the body's surface area.
- The chest equals 9% and the stomach equals 9% of the body's surface area.
- The upper back equals 9% and the lower back equals 9% of the body's surface area.
- The front and back of each leg and foot equal 18% of the body's surface area.
- The genital area equals 1% of the body's surface area.

II. Nursing Management:
A. Emergency or Resuscitation phase:

Assess patient's ABC (Airways, breathing and circulation).
Provide supplemental oxygen if necessary.
Restore fluids to avoid hypovolemic shock.
Monitor urine output, respiratory status, and cardiac monitoring if indicated.
Remove affected clothing and keep patient warm.
Assess neurologic status.

B. Resuscitative Phase:

Prevent hypovolemic shock by fluid replacement.
Use fluid resuscitation formula such as Modified Brooke, Parkland, or Modified Parkland.

C. Acute Phase:

Focus on wound care and pain control.
Monitor vital signs, peripheral pulses, fluid intake and output, cardiac rhythm, and pulmonary function.
Provide nutritional support and balanced restorative diet and drinks.
Focus on infection control, pain management, and physical therapy.

D. Rehabitative Phase:

Focus on restoring normal function.
Nurse's role to prepare patient for self-care after hospitalization.
Overlaps with the Acute Phase.

Case Study: A patient presents with a red area on the skin that does not change color with pressure. The area feels firm and warmer than the surrounding tissue.

What stage of pressure injury does this description most likely represent?

A) Stage 1

B) Stage 2

C) Stage 3

D) Stage 4

Correct Answer: A) Stage 1

Explanation:

A) Stage 1: This description matches Stage 1 pressure injury, where the skin is intact but exhibits redness that does not blanch.

B) Stage 2: Stage 2 involves partial loss of the dermis and presents as an ulcer or blister, not just redness.

C) Stage 3: Stage 3 involves full-thickness loss with visible subcutaneous tissue, which is not described here.

D) Stage 4: Stage 4 involves exposure of underlying structures such as bone or muscle, which is not indicated in the description.

Que: Which of the following statements by a nurse indicates proper management during the Emergency or Resuscitation phase for a burn patient?

A. "I'm closely monitoring the patient's urine output and assessing their neurologic status."

B. "I'm applying antibiotic ointment to the burn wounds for infection control."

C. "I'm using the Rule of Nines to assess the body surface area affected by burns."

D. "I'm administering pain medication to the patient for wound care."

E. "I'm instructing the patient on exercises to restore normal function."

Correct Answer: A

Explanation: During the Emergency or Resuscitation phase, it is essential for the nurse to assess the patient's ABC (Airways, breathing, and circulation) and monitor urine output, as well as assess the patient's neurologic status. These actions are critical for ensuring the patient's immediate well-being and detecting any potential complications. Option A is correct because it addresses these important aspects of care.

Option B is incorrect because applying antibiotic ointment is typically done during the Acute Phase, not the Emergency or Resuscitation phase.
Option C is incorrect because the Rule of Nines is used to assess the body surface area affected by burns, which is relevant to the assessment but not specific to the management in the Emergency or Resuscitation phase.
Option D is incorrect because administering pain medication is important for pain control but is more relevant to the Acute Phase of burn management.
Option E is incorrect because preparing the patient for self-care and instructing on exercises are part of the Rehabilitative Phase, which occurs later in the treatment process, not during the Emergency or Resuscitation phase.

Que : What is the purpose of elevating the extremities in burn injury management?

A. To prevent respiratory complications

B. To aid in shock prevention

C. To facilitate IV fluid administration

D. To support wound healing

Correct Answer: B

Explanation:

A (Incorrect): Elevating extremities does not directly prevent respiratory complications.

B (Correct): Elevating extremities helps prevent shock by promoting better circulation and fluid distribution in the body.

C (Incorrect): Elevating extremities is not related to the facilitation of IV fluid administration.

D (Incorrect): Although elevation might indirectly affect wound healing, its primary purpose in this context is to assist in shock prevention.

Case Study: A patient presents with a shallow ulcer with a red-pink base that resembles a blister filled with serum.

Which stage of pressure injury does this presentation most likely correspond to?

A) Stage 1

B) Stage 2

C) Stage 3

D) Stage 4

Correct Answer: B) Stage 2

Explanation:

A) Stage 1: Stage 1 is characterized by intact skin with redness, not an ulcer or blister.

B) Stage 2: Stage 2 is defined by partial-thickness loss of the dermis, presenting as a shallow ulcer with a red or pink base or a serum-filled blister.

C) Stage 3: Stage 3 involves full-thickness skin loss with visible subcutaneous tissue, which is not described here.

D) Stage 4: Stage 4 involves full-thickness loss with exposure of underlying structures, not a shallow ulcer or blister.

Que: A patient with a large burn wound is being treated with a skin covering that needs to be replaced every 2 to 5 days and is applied over granulation tissue. What type of dressing is being used?

a) Amniotic Membranes
b) Cultured Skin
c) Artificial Skin
d) Xenograft
e) Autograft

Right Answer: d) Xenograft

Explanation:

- **a) Amniotic Membranes**: Incorrect. These are typically replaced every 48 hours, not 2 to 5 days.

- **b) Cultured Skin**: Incorrect. Cultured skin is lab-grown and not replaced frequently; it's applied for permanent coverage.

- **c) Artificial Skin**: Incorrect. Artificial skin is a two-layer system that stays in place to support autografts rather than being replaced frequently.

- **d) Xenograft**: Correct. Xenograft, or heterograft, involves pigskin that is placed over granulation tissue and needs to be replaced every 2 to 5 days.

- **e) Autograft**: Incorrect. Autografts are taken from the patient's own body and provide permanent coverage; they are not replaced frequently.

Endocrine System

Practice Session

Que: A patient with Addison's disease reports feeling increasingly fatigued and has low blood pressure. They have recently been under a lot of stress.

What are the essential aspects of managing this patient's condition?

A) Administer glucocorticoid and mineralocorticoid medications

B) Increase fluid intake to manage low blood pressure

C) Monitor white blood cell count and electrolyte levels

D) Encourage high levels of physical activity

E) Avoid over-the-counter medications

Answer: A) Administer glucocorticoid and mineralocorticoid medications and C) Monitor white blood cell count and electrolyte levels

Explanation:

A) Administer glucocorticoid and mineralocorticoid medications is correct as these are necessary for managing Addison's disease.

B) Increase fluid intake to manage low blood pressure is less specific and not as targeted as medication for adrenal insufficiency.

C) Monitor white blood cell count and electrolyte levels is correct to ensure proper management and detect potential complications.

D) Encourage high levels of physical activity is not recommended due to the risk of exacerbating fatigue.

E) Avoid over-the-counter medications is generally good advice but not specific to the immediate management of Addison's disease.

Que: Which of the following is the most appropriate nursing intervention for a patient with Addison's disease experiencing an acute adrenal crisis?

A) Administering IV fluids containing dextrose

B) Administering high doses of glucocorticoids

C) Administering a potassium-sparing diuretic

D) Administering beta-adrenergic blockers

Explanation:

An acute adrenal crisis can occur when the patient experiences a sudden and severe worsening of symptoms due to stress or illness. Nursing management of a patient with Addison's disease during an acute adrenal crisis is critical, and it involves prompt intervention to prevent life-threatening complications.

A) Administering IV fluids containing dextrose: This option is partially correct as it addresses the fluid and electrolyte imbalances that can occur during an acute adrenal crisis. Addison's disease patients may experience hypotension, dehydration, and hyponatremia, which can be corrected with the administration of fluids containing dextrose. However, this option does not address the underlying cause of the crisis.

B) Administering high doses of glucocorticoids: This option is the correct answer as it addresses the underlying cause of the crisis, which is the lack of cortisol production. Patients with Addison's disease need lifelong replacement therapy with glucocorticoids, and during an acute adrenal crisis, high doses of glucocorticoids are necessary to prevent life-threatening complications such as hypotension, shock, and renal failure.

C) Administering a potassium-sparing diuretic: This option is incorrect as it does not address the underlying cause of the crisis. Potassium-sparing diuretics are used to treat hypertension and edema and can be harmful to patients with Addison's disease who are already experiencing electrolyte imbalances.

D) Administering beta-adrenergic blockers: This option is incorrect as it can worsen the patient's condition. Beta-adrenergic blockers are contraindicated in patients with Addison's disease as they can mask the signs and symptoms of hypoglycemia, which can be life-threatening in these patients. Furthermore, beta-adrenergic blockers can exacerbate the hypotension that occurs during an acute adrenal crisis.

Que: Ms. Jones, a 35-year-old woman, presents to the clinic with complaints of excessive thirst, frequent urination, and unexplained weight loss over the past few weeks. She reports feeling fatigued and irritable despite getting enough rest.

Which of the following statements from the patient reveals that she may have diabetes mellitus?

A) "I've been feeling more tired than usual lately."

B) "I've been experiencing some headaches occasionally."

C) "I've noticed that my hair seems to be falling out more."

D) "I've been drinking a lot of water and urinating frequently."

Answer: D

Explanation:

Option D: Excessive thirst and frequent urination are classic symptoms of diabetes mellitus, indicating hyperglycemia and polyuria.

Options A, B, and C may suggest general symptoms that could be related to various health issues but do not specifically point towards diabetes mellitus.

Que: Mrs. Agrima is a 45-year-old woman who has recently been diagnosed with Addison's disease. Mrs. Agrima's medical history includes a history of autoimmune disorders and she is currently taking corticosteroid medications for her autoimmune conditions.

Which of the following is NOT a symptom of Addison's disease?

A) Salt craving

B) Increased blood sugar

C) Electrolyte imbalances including high potassium and calcium and low sodium

D) Increased sexual performance

E) Fatigue and weakness

Correct answer: D

Rationale and explanation:

Option A, B, C, and E all match the symptoms of Addison's disease. It is important to note that Addison's disease is characterized by decreased sexual performance, not increased sexual performance.
In comparison, Cushing syndrome is characterized by hypersecretion of adrenocortical hormones and symptoms that are opposite of those seen in Addison's disease. Symptoms of Cushing syndrome include weight gain, round face, thin skin that bruises easily, purple stretch marks, and excess hair growth.

Respiratory System and Drugs

Practice Session

Case Study: A patient is receiving mechanical ventilation and the tidal volume is set to deliver 500 mL of air with each breath.

Que: What does the tidal volume setting on the ventilator refer to?

A) The total number of breaths delivered per minute

B) The volume of air the patient receives with each breath

C) The pressure needed to deliver a set tidal volume

D) The amount of oxygen concentration delivered to the patient

Answer: B) The volume of air the patient receives with each breath

Explanation:

A) The total number of breaths delivered per minute refers to the rate setting, not the tidal volume.

B) The volume of air the patient receives with each breath is the correct description of tidal volume.

C) The pressure needed to deliver a set tidal volume pertains to peak airway inspiratory pressure, not tidal volume.

D) The amount of oxygen concentration delivered to the patient is related to FiO2, not tidal volume.

Case Study: A 40-year-old male experiencing an asthma attack presents with restlessness, wheezing, and uses accessory muscles for breathing. His heart rate is elevated, and his oxygen levels are dropping.

What is the immediate priority intervention for this patient?

A) Administer peak flow test

B) Provide emotional support

C) Monitor for cyanosis

D) Administer bronchodilator

E) Educate about long-term asthma management

Correct Answer: D) Administer bronchodilator

Explanation:

A) Administer peak flow test: While useful, a peak flow test is not the immediate priority during an acute attack.

B) Provide emotional support: Emotional support is important but not the immediate priority during an asthma attack.

C) Monitor for cyanosis: Monitoring for cyanosis is important, but immediate breathing support takes precedence.

D) Administer bronchodilator: This is the immediate intervention to open the airways and provide relief from the attack.

E) Educate about long-term asthma management: Long-term management education is important, but this is not urgent during an active attack.

Que:

Case Study: A 35-year-old female is admitted with severe shortness of breath and chest tightness that has not improved with her usual asthma medications. Her oxygen levels continue to drop, and she is starting to show signs of respiratory distress.

What is the most likely diagnosis in this scenario?

A) Mild asthma

B) Severe asthma exacerbation

C) Status asthmaticus

D) COPD

E) Pulmonary embolism

Correct Answer: C) Status asthmaticus

Explanation:

A) Mild asthma: The symptoms described are far too severe for mild asthma.

B) Severe asthma exacerbation: Although severe, this diagnosis does not capture the refractory nature of the episode, which aligns with status asthmaticus.

C) Status asthmaticus: This condition involves a life-threatening asthma attack that is unresponsive to usual treatments, as described in the case.

D) COPD: COPD is a different chronic condition not related to this asthma episode.

E) Pulmonary embolism: While it causes shortness of breath, a pulmonary embolism has distinct features not related to an asthma attack.

Case Study: A 35-year-old patient arrives at the clinic complaining of shortness of breath, wheezing, and chest tightness that occur mostly after exercising. He reports that these episodes have become more frequent and last longer, though they often resolve with his inhaler.

MCQ: What is the most likely diagnosis for this patient?

A) Chronic bronchitis

B) Asthma

C) Pulmonary embolism

D) Congestive heart failure

Correct Answer: B) Asthma

Explanation:

A) Chronic bronchitis: Chronic bronchitis usually involves a persistent cough and mucus production over a long period, unlike the episodic nature of asthma.

B) Asthma: Asthma is the correct answer because the patient presents with classic symptoms such as wheezing, chest tightness, and breathlessness, which often worsen with physical activity.

C) Pulmonary embolism: This condition presents with sudden shortness of breath and chest pain, often with no wheezing.

D) Congestive heart failure: This typically involves fluid overload, leg swelling, and fatigue, which do not match the patient's symptoms.

Case Study: A 22-year-old woman with asthma has been experiencing frequent nighttime wheezing and shortness of breath despite using her rescue inhaler regularly.

MCQ: Which of the following interventions is the most appropriate next step in her treatment plan?

A) Increase her rescue inhaler usage

B) Prescribe a long-term inhaled corticosteroid

C) Advise the use of a peak flow meter to monitor lung function

D) Suggest daily antihistamine therapy

Correct Answer: B) Prescribe a long-term inhaled corticosteroid

Explanation:

A) Increase her rescue inhaler usage: Frequent use of a rescue inhaler indicates poor asthma control and requires additional management, not just increased use of the inhaler.

B) Prescribe a long-term inhaled corticosteroid: This is correct because inhaled corticosteroids are the standard for long-term management of asthma, especially for patients with frequent symptoms.

C) Advise the use of a peak flow meter: While helpful for monitoring, it does not directly address worsening control of asthma.

D) Suggest daily antihistamine therapy: Antihistamines help with allergies but are not first-line treatments for asthma management.

Case Study: A 35-year-old man presents with a persistent cough, night sweats, and weight loss. He mentions recently being in close contact with a friend diagnosed with tuberculosis (TB). His chest x-ray shows granulomas in the upper lobes, and his sputum test confirms Mycobacterium tuberculosis.

MCQ: What is the most likely reason the patient developed tuberculosis?

A) He consumed contaminated food.

B) He contracted it through airborne transmission from his friend.

C) He was infected by a mosquito bite.

D) He inherited it genetically from his parents.

Correct Answer: B) He contracted it through airborne transmission from his friend.

Explanation:

A) Incorrect. TB is not spread through food but through airborne droplets.

B) Correct. TB is primarily transmitted through the inhalation of airborne droplets when an infected person coughs or sneezes.

C) Incorrect. TB is not transmitted through insect bites.

D) Incorrect. TB is not inherited genetically; it is caused by an infection with Mycobacterium tuberculosis.

Que: Jane, a 45-year-old female, presents to the emergency department with complaints of severe shortness of breath, rapid breathing, and confusion. She has a history of pneumonia and recently underwent surgery for a fractured leg. On examination, she is found to have bilateral crackles on lung auscultation and low oxygen saturation levels. Arterial blood gas analysis reveals hypoxemia and respiratory alkalosis. Jane is diagnosed with Acute Respiratory Distress Syndrome (ARDS).

Which of the following ways of nursing management is not appropriate for a patient with Acute Respiratory Distress Syndrome (ARDS)?

A) High-flow oxygen therapy via nasal cannula

B) Mechanical ventilation with low tidal volumes

C) Prone positioning

D) Aggressive fluid resuscitation

E) Administration of corticosteroids

F) Strict fluid restriction

D) Aggressive fluid resuscitation

In ARDS, patients often experience fluid accumulation in the lungs due to increased permeability of the alveolar-capillary membrane. Aggressive fluid resuscitation can exacerbate pulmonary edema and worsen respiratory distress. Fluid management in ARDS is typically conservative, aiming to avoid fluid overload and manage fluid balance carefully.

The other options are generally appropriate for managing ARDS:

A) High-flow oxygen therapy via nasal cannula: While not the primary treatment for severe ARDS, it can be used in less severe cases or as a bridge to more advanced support.

B) Mechanical ventilation with low tidal volumes: This strategy is part of protective lung ventilation, which is designed to minimize ventilator-induced lung injury.

C) Prone positioning: This can improve oxygenation by enhancing ventilation-perfusion matching in the lungs.

E) Administration of corticosteroids: Corticosteroids can help reduce inflammation and improve outcomes in ARDS.

F) Strict fluid restriction: This helps to avoid exacerbating pulmonary edema and maintain a more manageable fluid balance.

Que: Sarah, a 35-year-old woman, presents to the emergency department with complaints of difficulty breathing, chest tightness, and coughing. She reports a history of asthma and allergies. Upon examination, the healthcare provider hears wheezing during expiration. Sarah's vital signs are within normal limits, but she appears anxious.

What is the primary significance of wheezing in respiratory assessment?

A) Indicates normal, healthy airflow through the smaller airways

B) Signals upper airway obstruction

C) Suggests fluid in the airways

D) Alerts to potential airway obstructions

E) Resonates over the large airways indicating upper respiratory tract abnormalities

Answer and Explanation:

Correct Answer: D) Alerts to potential airway obstructions

Explanation:

A) Incorrect. Vesicular breath sounds indicate normal, healthy airflow through the smaller airways and alveoli, not wheezing.

B) Incorrect. Stridor, not wheezing, is a harsh vibratory sound signaling upper airway obstruction.

C) Incorrect. Crackles, fine or coarse, suggest fluid in the airways, not wheezing.

D) Correct. Wheezing, characterized by a high-pitched whistling sound, alerts healthcare providers to potential airway obstructions, often associated with conditions like asthma, COPD, or bronchitis.

E) Incorrect. Bronchial breath sounds resonate over the large airways, but wheezing is not described as bronchial breath sounds.

Que : A patient with asthma is prescribed theophylline to manage their symptoms. The patient is experiencing gastric irritation as a side effect of the medication.
What is the nursing management approach to address the patient's gastric irritation?
A) Administer the medication via IV

B) Crush or break the medication

C) Administer the medication with food and educate the patient not to take it on an empty stomach

D) Administer the medication at irregular intervals

Right Answer: C) Administer the medication with food and educate the patient not to take it on an empty stomach
Rationale: Administering the medication with food and educating the patient not to take it on an empty stomach helps to protect the drug from the acidic environment of the stomach and minimizes the risk of gastric irritation.

Explanation: Theophylline is a bronchodilator that relaxes the smooth muscles in the bronchial airways and pulmonary blood vessels. It is used to treat symptoms of lung conditions that block the airways, such as emphysema or chronic bronchitis, and is taken orally. The drug can cause side effects such as gastric irritation, tachycardia, insomnia, restlessness, confusion, and dysrhythmias. To minimize the risk of gastric irritation, it is important to administer the medication with food and educate the patient not to take it on an empty stomach. The enteric coated tablet form of the medication is also designed to protect it from the acidic environment of the stomach and should not be crushed or broken while administered to the patient. The drug should also be given at regular intervals to achieve a normal therapeutic level, and patients taking the drug should avoid cigarettes, tea, coffee, and chocolate as they can worsen respiratory conditions. It is important to monitor for drug interactions, as theophylline should not be given with antibiotics like ciprofloxacin or cimetidine as they can disturb the absorption of the drug and increase the risk of toxicity. If theophylline is administered via IV, it should be done slowly via an infusion pump.

Nursing therapies

> **tip** There are several types of therapy available for mental health care, each with its unique approach and techniques. Milieu Therapy, for instance, emphasizes the social environment of an individual. In this therapy, a team comprising nurses, doctors, therapists, psychiatrists, and psychologists establishes meaningful relationships with the clients. Through interaction within a community setting, clients develop values such as self-awareness, self-confidence, and decent behavior.

Interpersonal Therapy (IPT), on the other hand, focuses on building a strong therapeutic relationship between the therapist and the client. This relationship creates a safe space for clients to express their feelings and receive support. IPT operates on three levels: supportive, re-educative, and reconstructive. At each level, clients engage in activities aimed at modifying their feelings and behaviors towards others, ultimately leading to greater emotional and social freedom.

Behavior Therapy encompasses a range of techniques designed to modify maladaptive behaviors. The primary goal is to reinforce desirable behaviors while eliminating unwanted ones. Techniques in behavior therapy draw from theories of classical conditioning and operant conditioning. Classical conditioning involves associating a conditioned stimulus (CS) with an unrelated unconditioned stimulus (US) to produce a conditioned response (CR). Techniques like desensitization and aversion therapy are examples of classical conditioning used to treat phobias and undesirable behaviors, respectively.

Operant conditioning, another facet of behavior therapy, employs punishment or reinforcement to increase desirable behaviors and decrease undesirable ones. For instance, modeling involves observing others' acceptable behaviors and emulating them to facilitate behavior change.

Cognitive Therapy is a short-term psychotherapy that centers on present thinking, behavior, and communication patterns. Unlike traditional psychotherapy, cognitive therapy focuses on correcting distorted perceptions and dysfunctional beliefs in the here and now. This approach is particularly effective in treating anxiety and depressive disorders by addressing negative thought patterns and promoting problem-solving skills.

Practice Session-Which of the following statements best describes Milieu Therapy in the context of therapeutic care?

A) Milieu Therapy involves altering behavior through classical conditioning techniques. B) Milieu Therapy focuses on correcting distorted concepts and dysfunctional beliefs. C) Milieu Therapy emphasizes building meaningful relationships with clients in a community setting. D) Milieu Therapy uses reinforcement to eliminate unwanted behaviors.

Correct Answer: C) Milieu Therapy emphasizes building meaningful relationships with clients in a community setting.

Explanation:

Milieu Therapy is a therapeutic approach that involves creating a supportive and therapeutic environment in which a team of healthcare professionals, including nurses, doctors, therapists, psychiatrists, and psychologists, develop meaningful relationships with clients. The goal is to facilitate the client's interaction within a community setting and help them develop values such as self-awareness, self-confidence, and decent behavior. This therapy does not primarily focus on altering behavior through conditioning techniques (Option A), correcting distorted concepts (Option B), or using reinforcement to eliminate unwanted behaviors (Option D).

Que : Mrs. B is a 45-year-old woman who has been experiencing symptoms of depression and anxiety. She has been struggling with negative thoughts and beliefs about herself and her ability to cope with life's challenges. Mrs. B's healthcare provider has recommended that she participate in cognitive therapy to help manage her symptoms.

Which of the following is a goal of cognitive therapy?

A. To reinforce desirable behaviors and eliminate unwanted ones

B. To develop a strong therapeutic relationship between the therapist and client

C. To correct distorted concepts and dysfunctional beliefs

D. To treat phobias and anxieties through desensitization

Correct Answer: C

Rationale:

Option A (to reinforce desirable behaviors and eliminate unwanted ones) is a goal of behavior therapy, not cognitive therapy. Option B (to develop a strong therapeutic relationship between the therapist and client) is a goal of interpersonal therapy, not cognitive therapy. Option D (to treat phobias and anxieties through desensitization) is a technique used in behavior therapy, specifically classical conditioning, not cognitive therapy. Option C (to correct distorted concepts and dysfunctional beliefs) is the most appropriate answer because it accurately describes a goal of cognitive therapy.

Explanation:

Cognitive therapy is a form of psychotherapy that aims to help individuals identify and modify negative thoughts and beliefs that may be contributing to their emotional distress. It focuses on present thinking, behavior, and communication rather than on past experiences and is oriented towards problem-solving. By correcting distorted concepts and dysfunctional beliefs, individuals may be better able to cope with life's challenges and manage their symptoms of anxiety and depression. Other types of therapy, such as behavior therapy and interpersonal therapy, may also be useful in managing mental health conditions, but they have different goals and focus on different aspects of the therapeutic process.

Que : Which of the following is NOT one of the levels of treatment in interpersonal therapy (IPT)?

A. Supportive level

B. Re-educative level

C. Reconstructive level

D. Aversive level

Correct Answer: D

Rationale:

Option A (supportive level) is a part of interpersonal therapy (IPT) and involves providing a supportive communication and environment in which the patient can express their feelings and make decisions. Option B (re-educative level) is also a part of IPT and involves the patient learning new ways of behavioral change through techniques such as cognitive restructuring and psychotherapy. Option C (reconstructive level) is also a part of IPT and involves emotional and cognitive restructuring in order to increase the patient's understanding of themselves and their emotions, leading to greater emotional and social freedom. Option D (aversive level) is not a part of interpersonal therapy (IPT) and is therefore the correct answer.

Explanation:

Interpersonal therapy (IPT) is a form of psychotherapy that focuses on improving communication and relationships in order to treat depression and other mental health issues. It consists of three levels of treatment: supportive, re-educative, and reconstructive. The supportive level involves providing a supportive communication and environment in which the patient can express their feelings and make decisions. The re-educative level involves the patient learning new ways of behavioral change through techniques such as cognitive restructuring and psychotherapy. The reconstructive level involves emotional and cognitive restructuring in order to increase the patient's understanding of themselves and their emotions, leading to greater emotional and social freedom. Aversive level is not a part of IPT and refers to pairing undesirable behavior with an aversive stimulus in order to decrease the frequency of that behavior.

Pediatric Nursing

Practice Session

Que : Mrs. Jones brings her 3-year-old son, Timmy, to the clinic because he has been vomiting for the past 12 hours. Upon assessment, the nurse notes that Timmy is alert but appears weak and dehydrated. His vomitus is yellow-green and has a sour smell. What should be the nurse's priority intervention for Timmy?

A. Administer an antiemetic medication

B. Assess the force of the vomiting

C. Monitor electrolyte levels

D. Provide oral rehydration therapy as tolerated and as prescribed

Answer: D. Provide oral rehydration therapy as tolerated and as prescribed

Explanation: The priority intervention for Timmy is to provide oral rehydration therapy as tolerated and as prescribed because the major concerns when a child is vomiting are the risk of dehydration, the loss of fluid and electrolytes, and the development of metabolic alkalosis. In addition, the nurse should monitor the character, amount, and frequency of vomiting, assess the force of the vomiting, and monitor electrolyte levels. Administering an antiemetic medication may be necessary but is not the priority intervention.

Que : A 7-year-old child was diagnosed with rubella (German measles) and has been admitted to the hospital. Which of the following statements regarding the patient needs nursing intervention or is either right or wrong?

A. Rubella is a common viral disease that has teratogenic effects on the fetus during the first trimester of pregnancy.

B. Rubella is transmitted by droplet and direct contact with an infected person.

C. The discrete red maculopapular rash starts on the face and rapidly spreads to the entire body.

D. Rash disappears within 3 days.

E. Rubella is not contagious and does not require isolation.

F. The patient may develop complications such as thrombocytopenia, encephalitis, and arthritis.

Options A, B, C, and F are correct.

Option A is correct because Rubella is a viral disease that has teratogenic effects on the fetus during the first trimester of pregnancy. Pregnant women who contract rubella can have babies with congenital rubella syndrome (CRS), which can cause a range of birth defects, including deafness, blindness, and heart defects.

Option B is correct because Rubella is transmitted by droplet and direct contact with an infected person. Therefore, the patient needs nursing intervention to prevent the spread of the disease to others. The patient should be placed in isolation until they are no longer contagious.

Option C is correct because the discrete red maculopapular rash starts on the face and rapidly spreads to the entire body. The rash may last for up to three days and is accompanied by fever, swollen glands, and joint pain.

Option F is correct because the patient may develop complications such as thrombocytopenia, encephalitis, and arthritis. Nursing interventions such as monitoring vital signs, administering medications, and providing supportive care can help prevent and manage these complications.

Option D is incorrect because the rash associated with rubella usually lasts for up to three days, not disappearing within three days.

Option E is incorrect because Rubella is highly contagious and requires isolation to prevent the spread of the disease to others.

In conclusion, the correct answers are A, B, C, and F. The patient with rubella needs nursing intervention to prevent the spread of the disease to others, monitor for and manage potential complications, and provide supportive care.

Patient's History: Sumitra, a pediatric patient, was admitted to the hospital with suspected rheumatic fever. She had been experiencing a fever for the past two days, and her parents noticed that she had a recent episode of pharyngitis.

Nurse's Notes: When obtaining Sumitra's history, the nurse considered which information was most important. The nurse took note of the patient's symptoms, including vomiting and dizziness for two days, lack of interest in food, and a recent episode of pharyngitis.

Physician Orders: Based on Sumitra's symptoms and history, the physician ordered tests to confirm the diagnosis of rheumatic fever. The physician also prescribed medication to manage the patient's symptoms and reduce inflammation.

Lab Values: Lab tests showed elevated levels of anti-streptolysin O (ASO) antibodies, which confirmed the diagnosis of rheumatic fever.

Que : What is the most important information for the nurse to consider when obtaining the patient's history for suspected rheumatic fever?

a) Lack of interest in food

b) A fever that started 2 days ago

c) A recent episode of pharyngitis

d) Vomiting and dizziness for 2 days

Explanation: The correct answer is c) A recent episode of pharyngitis. Group A streptococcus (GAS) infections of the pharynx are the precipitating cause of rheumatic fever. A recent episode of pharyngitis is the most important factor in establishing the diagnosis of rheumatic fever. Option b) is incorrect because fever is a common symptom in many illnesses and is not specific to rheumatic fever. Option a) is also incorrect because lack of interest in food can be seen in many illnesses and is not specific to rheumatic fever. Option d) is incorrect because vomiting and dizziness are not specific to rheumatic fever.

Que : Which of the following interventions are appropriate for managing GERD in infants?

A. Assess for signs of dehydration.

B. Provide small, frequent feedings with predigested formula.

C. Place the infant in the prone position during sleep.

D. Feed solids first, followed by liquids.

E. Avoid feeding the child fatty foods, chocolate, tomato products, carbonated liquids, fruit juices, citrus products, and spicy foods.

Answer: A and B. Options A and B are correct because assessing for signs of dehydration and providing small, frequent feedings with predigested formula are appropriate interventions for managing GERD in infants.

Options C, D, and E are incorrect because placing the infant in the prone position during sleep, feeding solids first followed by liquids, and avoiding certain foods are not appropriate interventions for managing GERD in infants. The infant should be placed in the supine position during sleep, with the head of the bed elevated, and the parents should be instructed to avoid certain foods if the infant is older than 1 year.

Que : A 6-year-old child is brought to the clinic with a nosebleed. The nurse should:

1. Panic and call for emergency assistance.
2. Have the child lie down on their back.
3. Assist the child to a sitting up and leaning forward position.
4. Apply pressure to the upper portion of the nose.

Answer: 3

Explanation: When a child has a nosebleed, it is important for the nurse to remain calm and keep the child calm and quiet. Panic can cause the child to become agitated and difficult to cooperate. The child should be assisted to a sitting up and leaning forward position to prevent aspiration of blood. The child should not be placed in a lying down position because of the risk of aspiration. Nosebleeds usually originate in the anterior part of the nasal septum and can be controlled by applying pressure to the soft lower portion of the nose with the thumb and forefinger for at least 10 minutes. Therefore, option 4 is incorrect as it suggests applying pressure to the upper portion of the nose. Option 2 is also incorrect as it advises lying down. Finally, option 1 is incorrect as it suggests panic, which is not an appropriate response. Option 3 is the correct answer because it advises assisting the child to a sitting up and leaning forward position to prevent aspiration of blood.

Gerontology /Geriatric Nursing

NGN Case Study

1. History and Nurse Notes:

Mrs. Margaret Thompson, an 80-year-old female, is admitted to the medical-surgical unit with complaints of generalized weakness, shortness of breath, and confusion. She has a medical history of hypertension, type 2 diabetes, and osteoarthritis. The patient lives alone, and her daughter brought her to the hospital.

Nurse Notes:

Upon admission, Mrs. Thompson appeared fatigued and disoriented.

Blood pressure: 160/90 mmHg, Heart rate: 98 bpm, Respiratory rate: 22 bpm, Temperature: 99.2°F.

Mrs. Thompson has difficulty recalling recent events, and her daughter reports a decline in overall cognitive function over the past few weeks.

The patient complains of joint pain and stiffness in her knees.

Medication reconciliation reveals she is taking metformin, lisinopril, and ibuprofen for arthritis.

2. Medications:

a) Metformin (Glucophage):

Purpose: To manage type 2 diabetes.

Dosage: 1000 mg orally twice a day.

Side effects: GI upset, lactic acidosis (rare).

b) Lisinopril (Prinivil):

Purpose: To control hypertension.

Dosage: 10 mg orally once daily.

Side effects: Cough, hypotension.

c) Ibuprofen (Advil):

Purpose: To alleviate arthritis pain.

Dosage: 200 mg orally every 6 hours as needed.

Side effects: GI bleeding, renal impairment.

3. Vital Signs:

Blood Pressure: 150/85 mmHg

Heart Rate: 92 bpm

Respiratory Rate: 20 bpm

Temperature: 98.8°F

Oxygen Saturation: 95%

4. Lab Reports:

Fasting glucose: 160 mg/dL (elevated).

HbA1c: 8.5% (poorly controlled diabetes).

Blood Urea Nitrogen (BUN): 28 mg/dL (elevated).

Serum Creatinine: 1.5 mg/dL (elevated).

C-reactive protein (CRP): 15 mg/L (elevated).

Que What is a potential concern in managing pain for older adults with arthritis, especially those with hypertension?

a) Increased risk of cognitive decline

b) Adverse effects on renal function

c) Improved cardiovascular health

d) Enhanced joint mobility

Ans :

Explanation:

Correct Answer: b) Adverse effects on renal function

Arthritis pain management often involves nonsteroidal anti-inflammatory drugs (NSAIDs), which may pose a risk to renal function, especially in older adults with hypertension. NSAIDs can lead to fluid retention and increased blood pressure, potentially exacerbating hypertension and causing renal impairment.

Incorrect Options:

a) Increased risk of cognitive decline

While chronic pain may impact cognitive function, the primary concern with arthritis pain management in this case is related to renal function due to the use of NSAIDs.

c) Improved cardiovascular health

Pain management strategies may impact cardiovascular health indirectly, but the primary focus is on potential adverse effects on renal function, not cardiovascular improvement.

d) Enhanced joint mobility

While the goal of arthritis management is to improve joint mobility, the Que specifically addresses concerns related to hypertension and pain management. The use of NSAIDs and their potential impact on renal function is the primary concern in this context.

Que : Which of the following side effects should the nurse be particularly vigilant for in this case? (Select two options)

a) Gastrointestinal bleeding

b) Increased blood glucose levels

c) Renal impairment

d) Cough

e) Cognitive decline

f) Enhanced joint mobility

Ans :

Explanation:

Correct Answers: a) Gastrointestinal bleeding and c) Renal impairment

Gastrointestinal bleeding (a): NSAIDs, commonly prescribed for arthritis, can increase the risk of gastrointestinal bleeding. Monitoring for symptoms such as black stools or abdominal pain is crucial.

Renal impairment (c): NSAIDs, including those used for arthritis, may impact renal function. Regular monitoring of renal function is essential to detect any signs of impairment, such as changes in BUN and serum creatinine levels.

Incorrect Options:

b) Increased blood glucose levels

Arthritis medications, particularly NSAIDs, are not known to significantly affect blood glucose levels. This side effect is less relevant in this context.

d) Cough

Cough is a potential side effect of medications like ACE inhibitors, commonly used for hypertension. However, it is not directly related to arthritis medications in this case.

e) Cognitive decline

While cognitive decline may be a concern in elderly patients, it is not a common side effect of arthritis medications. This option is less relevant in the context of Mr. Johnson's case.

f) Enhanced joint mobility

Enhanced joint mobility is a desired outcome of arthritis management. It is not a side effect but a positive effect of appropriate treatment. This option is incorrect in the context of potential side effects.

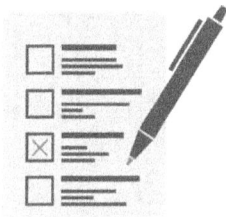

Practice Session

Que : Mrs. Vimal is a 78-year-old female who was admitted to the hospital with complaints of severe pain in her left hip. She has a history of hypertension and osteoarthritis. The physician has ordered analgesics to manage her pain. The nurse is reviewing Mrs. Vimal's medications and medical history to ensure that she does not receive any medications that could potentially cause harm.

Which of the following statements from the nurse indicates that she has a good understanding of medications to avoid in the older client?

A) "I will administer indomethacin to Mrs. Vimal for her hip pain."

B) "Ketorolac is a safe NSAID to give to older clients."

C) "Meperidine can cause confusion and is not recommended for older adults."

D) "Tricyclic antidepressants are a good option for treating depression in older clients."

E) "First-generation antihistamines are safe to use in older adults."

F) "Alpha1-blockers and centrally acting alpha2-agonists are safe for older adults with hypertension."

G) "Oxybutynin and tolterodine are effective medications for treating urge incontinence in older adults."
H) "Barbiturates and benzodiazepines are safe to use as sedative-hypnotics in older adults."

Answer:

The correct answers is C.

Explanation:

A) "I will administer indomethacin to Mrs. Vimal for her hip pain." - This statement is incorrect as indomethacin is a NSAID that should be avoided in older adults due to its potential to cause gastrointestinal bleeding, ulcers, and kidney damage.

B) "Ketorolac is a safe NSAID to give to older clients." - This statement is incorrect as ketorolac is also a NSAID that should be avoided in older adults due to its potential to cause kidney damage and gastrointestinal bleeding.

C) "Meperidine can cause confusion and is not recommended for older adults." - This statement is correct as meperidine is a medication that can cause confusion, delirium, and other adverse effects in older adults due to its metabolites accumulating in the body.

D) "Tricyclic antidepressants are a good option for treating depression in older clients." - This statement is incorrect as first-generation tricyclic antidepressants can cause several adverse effects, including anticholinergic effects, orthostatic hypotension, and cardiac arrhythmias, which can be dangerous for older adults.

E) "First-generation antihistamines are safe to use in older adults." - This statement is incorrect as first-generation antihistamines can cause sedation, confusion, and other adverse effects in older adults, increasing the risk of falls and accidents.

F) "Alpha1-blockers and centrally acting alpha2-agonists are safe for older adults with hypertension." - This statement is incorrect as both medications can cause orthostatic hypotension, dizziness, and falls, which can be dangerous for older adults.

G) "Oxybutynin and tolterodine are effective medications for treating urge incontinence in older adults." - This statement is incorrect as both medications can cause anticholinergic effects, dry mouth, constipation, and confusion, which can be dangerous for older adults.

H) "Barbiturates and benzodiazepines are safe to use as sedative-hypnotics in older adults." - This statement is incorrect as both medications can cause sedation, confusion, falls, respiratory depression, and other adverse effects in older adults, which can be life-threatening.

Nervous System/ Diseases

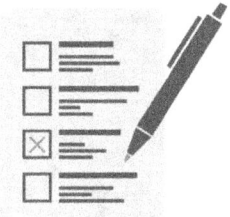

Practice Session

Which symptom would most likely indicate Bell's Palsy?

A. Severe muscle weakness and atrophy

B. Intense facial pain and sensitivity

C. Flaccid facial muscles and inability to close the eyelid

D. Tremors that improve with movement E. Difficulty breathing and speaking

Correct Answer: C. Flaccid facial muscles and inability to close the eyelid

Explanation:

A. Severe muscle weakness and atrophy: More characteristic of ALS.

B. Intense facial pain and sensitivity: Seen in Trigeminal Neuralgia.

C. Flaccid facial muscles and inability to close the eyelid: Typical of Bell's Palsy, resulting from paralysis on one side of the face.

D. Tremors that improve with movement: Associated with Parkinson's Disease.

E. Difficulty breathing and speaking: More relevant to ALS or Guillain-Barre Syndrome.

Que: Which of the following is a characteristic finding in the cerebrospinal fluid (CSF) of a patient with Guillain-Barre Syndrome?

A. Elevated gamma globulin levels

B. Decreased protein levels

C. Increased white blood cell count

D. Elevated protein levels with normal white blood cell count

E. Normal glucose levels

Correct Answer: D. Elevated protein levels with normal white blood cell count

Explanation:

A. Elevated gamma globulin levels: This is a feature of Multiple Sclerosis.

B. Decreased protein levels: Not typical of Guillain-Barre Syndrome.

C. Increased white blood cell count: This is seen in bacterial meningitis or encephalitis, not Guillain-Barre Syndrome.

D. Elevated protein levels with normal white blood cell count: This is characteristic of Guillain-Barre Syndrome.

E. Normal glucose levels: Not specific to Guillain-Barre Syndrome; glucose levels are typically normal in Guillain-Barre.

8. What is an appropriate management strategy for a patient experiencing double vision (diplopia) due to Multiple Sclerosis (MS)?

A. Administer anticholinesterase medications

B. Use an eye patch

C. Avoid extreme temperatures in food and fluids

D. Encourage frequent rest periods

E. Perform facial exercises

Correct Answer: B. Use an eye patch

Explanation:

A. Administer anticholinesterase medications: This is for Myasthenia Gravis, not MS.

B. Use an eye patch: This helps manage double vision in MS.

C. Avoid extreme temperatures in food and fluids: This is relevant to Trigeminal Neuralgia.

D. Encourage frequent rest periods: Helpful for general fatigue but not specific to managing double vision in MS.

E. Perform facial exercises: Relevant for Bell's Palsy.

Que: Which factor is least likely to trigger an exacerbation in Multiple Sclerosis (MS)?

A. Stress

B. Overheating

C. Pregnancy

D. Low-fat diet

E. Infection

Correct Answer: D. Low-fat diet

Explanation:

A. Stress: Known to trigger exacerbations in MS.

B. Overheating: Can worsen MS symptoms.

C. Pregnancy: Can influence the course of MS.

D. Low-fat diet: While a balanced diet is important, a low-fat diet is not specifically known to trigger MS exacerbations.

E. Infection: Can trigger MS flare-ups.

Que : Which of the following statements from the nurse indicates that they understand the significance of the Babinski reflex?

A) "The Babinski reflex is a normal reflex in adults."

B) "The Babinski reflex is elicited by touching the back of the throat."

C) "The Babinski reflex indicates a dysfunction of cranial nerve V."

D) "The Babinski reflex is elicited by firmly stroking the lateral aspect of the sole of the foot."

E) "The Babinski reflex is a sign of a healthy central nervous system."

F) "The Babinski reflex is a sign of dysfunction of cranial nerves IX and X."

G) "The Babinski reflex is only present in infants."

H) "The Babinski reflex is a sign of peripheral nervous system disease."

Correct answers: D, H, and E

Explanation:

The Babinski reflex, or Babinski sign, is a reflex action seen when the underside of the foot is stroked with a blunt instrument. In infants, this reflex is expected and manifests as an upward movement of the big toe with the other toes spreading out. This reaction is due to the still-developing nervous system in young children and typically fades by age 2.

In contrast, the Babinski reflex is unusual in adults and may signal a neurological issue. Its presence in adults can indicate a dysfunction in the corticospinal tract, which plays a key role in motor control.

Option A is incorrect because the Babinski reflex is not normal in adults. Option B is incorrect because the reflex being referred to in the statement is actually the Gag reflex, not the Babinski reflex. Option C is incorrect because the Babinski reflex indicates a dysfunction of the central nervous system, not cranial nerve V. Option D is correct because this is an accurate statement about how to elicit the Babinski reflex. Option E is correct because the Babinski reflex is indeed a sign of a healthy central nervous system in infants while in adults it can indicate some abnormality in central nervous system. Option F is incorrect because the reflex being referred to in the statement is actually the Gag reflex, not the Babinski reflex. Option G is incorrect because the Babinski reflex can also be present in adults with certain central nervous system disorders. Option H is correct because the Babinski reflex is a sign of peripheral nervous system disease.

Que : Which of the following statements from the patient indicates that they may have an epidural hematoma?

A. "I have been experiencing headaches and dizziness since my fall."

B. "My vision has been blurry since I hit my head."

C. "I have a bump on my forehead where I hit my head."

D. "I lost consciousness for a few minutes after I fell."

Answer: D. "I lost consciousness for a few minutes after I fell."

Explanation: The passage describes that epidural hematoma is often associated with temporary loss of consciousness, followed by a lucid period that then rapidly progresses to coma. Therefore, a patient who has lost consciousness for a few minutes after a head injury is more likely to have an epidural hematoma than the other options.

Option A is incorrect because headaches and dizziness can be associated with many types of head injuries, not just epidural hematomas.

Option B is incorrect because blurry vision is not specifically associated with epidural hematomas, and could be a symptom of other head injuries or conditions.

Option C is incorrect because a bump on the forehead indicates a superficial injury and does not provide information about potential brain injury.

Que: A nurse is caring for a client with a spinal cord injury who develops autonomic dysreflexia. Which of the following statements said by the nurse indicates that they understand the appropriate management of this condition?

Option A: "I will wait and see if the client's symptoms resolve on their own."

Option B: "I will administer a stimulant laxative to help with constipation."

Option C: "I will administer an antihypertensive medication immediately."

Option D: "I will assess for bladder distention and remove any noxious stimuli."

Option E: "I will check the client's oxygen saturation and provide supplemental oxygen if needed."
Option F: "I will assess the client's skin for pressure ulcers."

Correct answers: D

Explanation:

Autonomic dysreflexia is a medical emergency that can occur in individuals with spinal cord injuries. It is characterized by severe hypertension, bradycardia, severe headache, nasal stuffiness, and flushing, and is typically caused by a noxious stimulus, such as bladder distention or constipation. The prompt removal of the noxious stimulus is crucial to prevent further complications, such as hypertensive stroke.

The nurse should first assess for bladder distention and remove any noxious stimuli. If the client has a urinary catheter, the nurse should check for kinks in the tubing. Additionally, if the nurse suspects fecal impaction, they should disimpact the client if necessary. Option A is incorrect because waiting for the client's symptoms to resolve on their own could be dangerous and increase the risk of complications. Option B is incorrect because administering a stimulant laxative would not address the underlying cause of autonomic dysreflexia. Option C is incorrect because administering an antihypertensive medication should only be done under the guidance of a healthcare provider. Option E is incorrect because checking the client's oxygen saturation and providing supplemental oxygen is not the first priority in managing autonomic dysreflexia. Option F is incorrect because assessing the client's skin for pressure ulcers is not relevant to managing autonomic dysreflexia.

Que: Saigrace is a 25-year-old male who presents to the emergency department with a fever, headache, and neck stiffness. He reports feeling lethargic and having difficulty with bright lights. Upon examination, Kernig's sign and Brudzinski's sign are positive. A lumbar puncture is performed, and the CSF analysis shows cloudy fluid with increased protein, increased white blood cells, and decreased glucose counts. Based on these findings, Saigrace is diagnosed with meningitis.

Which of the following statements of the patient indicates that Saigrace has meningitis?

A. Saigrace reports feeling lethargic.

B. Saigrace has positive Kernig's sign and Brudzinski's sign.

C. Saigrace has a red, macular rash.

D. Saigrace complains of abdominal pain.

E. Saigrace has a chest pain.

F. Saigrace has a history of sinus infections.

Correct answers: B

Explanation:

B. Saigrace having positive Kernig's sign and Brudzinski's sign indicates meningeal irritation, which is a characteristic sign of meningitis.

Option A is incorrect because lethargy is a common symptom in many conditions and is not specific to meningitis. Option C is incorrect because a red, macular rash is a sign of meningococcal meningitis, which is a specific type of meningitis and not present in all cases. Option D and E are incorrect because abdominal and chest pain are not characteristic signs of meningitis. Option F is incorrect because a history of sinus infections is a predisposing factor, but not a definitive indicator, of meningitis

Seizure

> **tip** Seizures or epilepsy occur due to abnormal and excessive electrical discharge in the brain that disturbs normal functioning.

Seizures are broadly divided into Generalized seizures and Partial seizures.

Generalized seizures involve abnormal electrical activity in both cerebral hemispheres and are usually caused by genetic or metabolic disorders. Absence seizures, tonic-clonic seizures, and myoclonic seizures are all types of generalized seizures.

Absence seizures last for a short time and are common in children. Tonic-clonic seizures involve repetition of the tonic and clonic phase of the seizure. Myoclonic seizures involve short jerking of body parts, and atonic seizures cause a brief and sudden loss of muscle tone.

Partial seizures are divided into simple partial and complex partial seizures. Simple partial seizures originate on one side of the brain and spread to other areas. Complex partial seizures begin in an area of the brain that affects consciousness.

Nursing interventions for seizures include making the patient lie down, managing ABC or airways breathing and circulation, tilting the patient's head to take out secretions, and identifying the type and pattern of seizure to identify the treatment approach.

The main antiseizure medications are Carbamazepine, Phenytoin, Lorazepam, Gabapentin, Pregabalin, Phenobarbital, and Clonazepam.

These medications should be used with care or continuously monitored for patients who are on antipsychotic or anticoagulants medications like warfarin already. Supplements, milk, and antacids can interfere with absorption, so the patient should not take these when anti-seizure medicines are given.

Phenytoin is used to treat tonic-clonic and partial seizures and can cause side effects like swelling and bleeding of the gums, headache, nausea, vomiting, constipation, dizziness, feeling of spinning, drowsiness, trouble sleeping, or nervousness.

Nursing interventions for patients taking phenytoin include taking good care of oral hygiene and oral health, understanding that it can decrease the efficiency of birth control pills, and avoiding the drug if the woman is pregnant as it is a category D medication that may harm the growing fetus.

Which of the following statements by a nurse indicates a correct nursing intervention for managing seizures in a hospital setting?

A) "It's important to elevate the patient's head during a seizure."

B) "Patients can take supplements along with their antiseizure medications."

C) "Phenytoin is safe for pregnant women to use during seizures."

D) "Gabapentin is commonly used to treat absence seizures."

E) "Patients on antipsychotic medications don't need monitoring when taking antiseizure drugs."

Correct Answer: A) "It's important to elevate the patient's head during a seizure."
Explanation: Elevating the patient's head during a seizure is a correct nursing intervention to help manage the airway and prevent aspiration. This statement aligns with proper seizure management procedures.
Explanation for Incorrect Options:
B) "Patients can take supplements along with their antiseizure medications." - This is incorrect because supplements can interfere with the absorption of antiseizure medications, so patients should not take them together.
C) "Phenytoin is safe for pregnant women to use during seizures." - This is incorrect because phenytoin is classified as a category D medication, which means it may harm the growing fetus, so it should be avoided during pregnancy.
D) "Gabapentin is commonly used to treat absence seizures." - This is incorrect because gabapentin is not typically used to treat absence seizures; it is more commonly used for other types of seizures.
E) "Patients on antipsychotic medications don't need monitoring when taking antiseizure drugs." - This is incorrect because patients on antipsychotic medications should be continuously monitored when taking antiseizure drugs due to potential interactions between the medications.

Which of the following statement of a patient indicates that they need immediate nursing intervention for seizure management?
A) "I occasionally experience short jerking of my body parts."

B) "I often have a brief and sudden loss of muscle tone."

C) "I have been taking antacids regularly."

D) "I am currently pregnant and taking phenytoin."

E) "I have a family history of epilepsy."

Correct Answer: D) "I am currently pregnant and taking phenytoin."

Explanation: A) This statement describes myoclonic seizures, which may require intervention but are not an immediate concern. B) This statement describes atonic seizures, which may require intervention but are not an immediate concern. C) Taking antacids may interfere with antiseizure medication absorption but does not indicate an immediate need for nursing intervention. D) This statement indicates that the patient is pregnant and taking phenytoin, which is a category D medication that may harm the fetus. This requires immediate nursing intervention to assess and potentially adjust the medication regimen. E) Family history of epilepsy is not an immediate indicator for nursing intervention.

Parkinson's Disease

> **tip** Parkinson's disease is a neural degenerative disorder that causes unintended or uncontrollable movements, such as shaking, stiffness, and difficulty with balance and coordination, caused by depleted dopamine levels.
> Symptoms include slow and sluggish movement (bradykinesia), loss of coordination, jerking or tremors in hands and fingers, monotonous speech, and facial expression.
> Nursing interventions involve maintaining physical coordination, posture, and rehabilitative approach with physical therapy, promoting slow walking and maintaining posture while sitting, promoting independence in performing ADLs, achieving optimal bowel elimination, attaining and maintaining acceptable nutritional status, achieving effective communication, and developing positive coping mechanisms.
> Medical interventions may include medications that increase dopamine levels, deep brain stimulation, and surgery.

In managing a patient with Parkinson's disease, which of the following habits of the patient needs to be emphasized for their care? Select two correct options from the list below:

Options:

A) Regularly practicing high-intensity exercises

B) Consuming a diet rich in antioxidants

C) Prioritizing adequate sleep and rest

D) Avoiding all forms of physical activity

E) Limiting fluid intake to prevent urinary incontinence

F) Reducing the intake of dopamine-inhibiting foods

G) Practicing relaxation techniques and stress management

H) Completely avoiding medications to prevent side effects

Explanation:

B) Consuming a diet rich in antioxidants: Antioxidants can help protect neurons and may have a neuroprotective effect, making this an important aspect of managing Parkinson's disease.

C) Prioritizing adequate sleep and rest: Proper sleep and rest are crucial for overall well-being and can help manage symptoms associated with Parkinson's disease. Sleep disturbances are common in Parkinson's patients, so emphasizing good sleep hygiene is important.

G) Practicing relaxation techniques and stress management: Stress management techniques can be beneficial for Parkinson's patients, as stress can exacerbate symptoms.

Incorrect:

A) Regularly practicing high-intensity exercises: While exercise is beneficial for Parkinson's patients, high-intensity exercises may not always be suitable. It's important to tailor exercise programs to the individual's capabilities and needs.
D) Avoiding all forms of physical activity: This is incorrect. Physical activity, within the patient's capabilities, is generally encouraged for Parkinson's patients.
E) Limiting fluid intake to prevent urinary incontinence: Limiting fluid intake is not a recommended strategy for managing Parkinson's disease. Proper hydration is important for overall health.
F) Reducing the intake of dopamine-inhibiting foods: This is not a standard recommendation for managing Parkinson's disease. Medications are typically used to address dopamine levels.
H) Completely avoiding medications to prevent side effects: Avoiding medications is not a recommended approach for managing Parkinson's disease. Medications are often prescribed to alleviate symptoms and manage the condition.

Musculo-Skeletal System /Drugs

Gout and Management

Gout manifests when there is an accumulation of uric acid in the bloodstream, resulting in the deposition of urate crystals within the joints. This condition progresses through distinct phases: Asymptomatic, Acute, Intermittent, and Chronic, each characterized by varying degrees of symptom severity and duration. Tophi, chalky deposits of urate crystals, serve as a common hallmark of gout, aiding in its identification.

Symptoms of gout encompass joint pain, skin rashes, and the formation of renal stones, contributing to significant discomfort and impaired mobility for affected individuals. Managing gout necessitates dietary modifications, including the avoidance of protein-rich and purine-containing foods, coupled with increased consumption of alkaline vegetables and water.

Pharmacological interventions for gout encompass nonsteroidal anti-inflammatory drugs (NSAIDs), probenecid, allopurinol, and colchicine. Probenecid usage should be cautious with aspirin due to the potential risk of elevated uric acid levels. Allopurinol administration may lead to visual changes and should not be combined with hypoglycemic agents, warfarin, or citrus fruits, which can exacerbate symptoms.

Nursing considerations in gout management entail vigilant monitoring for adverse medication effects, patient education regarding lifestyle adjustments, and encouragement of adequate hydration.

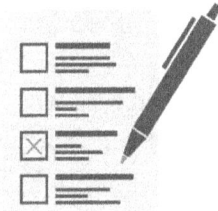

Practice Session

In nursing management of gout, which of the following are important nursing considerations for patients?
Options:

A) Encouraging smoking cessation

B) Monitoring renal function regularly

C) Advising patients to consume protein-rich foods

D) Recommending high-fructose corn syrup intake

E) Promoting alcohol consumption for pain relief

F) Collaborating with cardiologists for care coordination

G) Administering NSAIDs without monitoring

Correct Answers: B) Monitoring renal function regularly and F) Collaborating with dietitians for care coordination.

Explanation: B) Monitoring renal function regularly: This is an important nursing consideration for patients with gout because some medications used for gout management can affect renal function. Regular monitoring helps detect and manage any renal impairment promptly.

F) Collaborating with dietitians for care coordination: Collaborating with dietitians is crucial in gout management because dietary changes are a key part of the treatment plan. Dietitians can provide guidance on avoiding purine-containing foods and making appropriate dietary modifications to prevent gout exacerbations.

A) Encouraging smoking cessation: While smoking cessation is important for overall health, it is not a specific nursing consideration directly related to gout management.

C) Advising patients to consume protein-rich foods: Gout management typically involves avoiding protein-rich foods, so advising patients to consume them would not be appropriate.

D) Recommending high-fructose corn syrup intake: High-fructose corn syrup can increase uric acid levels, which can exacerbate gout. Recommending its intake would not be a suitable nursing consideration.

E) Promoting alcohol consumption for pain relief: Alcohol consumption can trigger gout attacks, so promoting its consumption for pain relief is not advisable.

G) Administering NSAIDs without monitoring: While NSAIDs may be used in gout management, administering them without monitoring for adverse effects is not a safe nursing practice. Monitoring for side effects is essential.

Que : Mrs. Agrima is a 67-year-old woman who has been diagnosed with gout. She has been experiencing pain and inflammation in her toes for the past few weeks and has been prescribed NSAIDs for pain management. However, she is also taking aspirin for her heart condition and is concerned about the potential interactions between the two medications.

Which of the following statements is true regarding the use of probenecid in patients with gout?

A) Probenecid should be avoided in patients taking aspirin

B) Probenecid can cause visual disturbances in some patients

C) Probenecid can increase the risk of extreme bleeding if taken with warfarin

D) Probenecid should not be taken with citrus fruits

Correct answer: A

Rationale:

Option A is correct because probenecid should never be used with aspirin as salicylates can cause elevation of the uric acid. For B, Probenecid is not commonly associated with visual disturbances.. Option

C is incorrect because it refers to allopurinol, not probenecid. Option D is incorrect because it also refers to allopurinol, not probenecid.

Explanation:

It is important for healthcare professionals to be aware of the potential interactions and side effects of medications used to treat gout in order to ensure the safe and effective management of the disease. Probenecid is a medication used to treat gout, but it should not be used in conjunction with aspirin due to the potential for salicylates to cause an elevation of uric acid levels. Allopurinol, on the other hand, can cause visual disturbances in some patients and should not be taken with hypoglycemic agents or citrus fruits. It is also important to be aware of the potential for allopurinol to increase the effects of warfarin, which can lead to extreme bleeding.

Osteoarthritis

Osteoarthritis stands as the prevailing arthritis condition affecting the elderly demographic. It stems from the gradual deterioration of protective cartilage, primarily found in weight-bearing joints like the hands, knees, hips, and spine.

Manifestations of osteoarthritis encompass physical symptoms such as Heberden's nodes or Bouchard's nodes in the hands. Heberden's nodes emerge as small bony growths at the finger joint nearest to the tip, while Bouchard's nodes manifest at the middle joint of the finger.

The hallmark symptom of osteoarthritis remains joint pain, escalating as the condition advances. Initially experienced during movement and activity, the pain extends to resting periods as the disease progresses. Swelling exacerbates discomfort, particularly in extreme temperature and humidity conditions.

Treatment strategies for osteoarthritis revolve around pain management and inflammation reduction. Modalities include topical pain-relieving creams like acetaminophen and NSAIDs, along with hot and cold therapy and splint devices to alleviate inflammation. Steroid therapy and corticosteroid injections into affected joints constitute common treatments. In severe instances, surgical interventions such as osteotomy or hip and knee replacements may be necessary.

Rest assumes paramount importance for osteoarthritis patients, who should refrain from using high pillows under their knees or heads. Maintaining a healthy weight and adhering to a balanced diet prove essential to alleviate pressure on the knees and hips. Light exercise aids in improving mobility and reducing joint stiffness, although rigorous exercises should be avoided to prevent additional stress on affected joints.

Que: Mr. Alvin is a 65-year-old man who has been diagnosed with osteoarthritis. He is experiencing joint pain and swelling in his hands and knees, and has difficulty performing everyday activities due to the pain. Mr. Alvin's doctor has prescribed acetaminophen and hot and cold therapy for pain management, and has recommended that he take rest and maintain a healthy weight.

Which of the following is a treatment option for severe osteoarthritis?

A. Osteotomy

B. Corticosteroid injection

C. Heat pads

D. Hip and knee replacement

Correct answer: D

Rationale: Osteoarthritis is a chronic condition that results from the wear and tear of the protective cartilage in the joints. It most commonly affects the hands, knees, hips, and spine and can cause joint pain, swelling, and stiffness. The treatment approach for osteoarthritis is to manage the pain and reduce inflammation, which can be achieved through the use of pain relieving creams, hot and cold therapy, and splint devices. In severe cases, corticosteroid injection and surgical interventions such as osteotomy or hip and knee replacement may be used. It is important for patients with osteoarthritis to take rest, maintain a healthy weight, and engage in light exercises to reduce joint stiffness and improve movement.

Option D is correct because hip and knee replacement is a treatment option for severe osteoarthritis. Option A is incorrect because osteotomy is a surgical intervention that may be used to correct deformed joints, but is not necessarily used for severe osteoarthritis. Option B is incorrect because corticosteroid injection is a treatment option for intense pain, but is not necessarily used for severe osteoarthritis. Option C is incorrect because heat pads are a treatment option for pain management, but are not necessarily used for severe osteoarthritis.

Rheumatoid arthritis

Rheumatoid Arthritis is an autoimmune inflammatory condition of joints.
Autoimmune disease is when the body's natural defense system mistakenly attacks normal cells.
In Rheumatoid Arthritis, there is destruction of the synovial membrane and connective tissues of the joint.
The development of Rheumatoid Arthritis involves inflammation of the joints, followed by the formation of fibrous tissue (pannus) between the synovial tissue and articular cartilage, which gradually destroys the space in between the joints and causes bones to fuse.
Symptoms include difficulty in movement of bones, crooked or curved appearance of both hands and feet, feverishness, and long-lasting symptoms.

Assessment of Rheumatoid Arthritis:

In Rheumatoid Arthritis, joints feel soft on touch and there are episodes of morning stiffness with pain that last for about an hour.
There may be symmetric crooked appearance of hands and feet.
Blood tests show positive rheumatoid factor and increased ESR.
Medical Treatment for Rheumatoid Arthritis:

There is no cure for Rheumatoid Arthritis, but treatment can improve symptoms.
NSAIDs such as ibuprofen are commonly used to reduce pain and inflammation.
Steroids such as Prednisone or dexamethasone can also be used, but may cause severe hyperglycemia.
Gold Salts are another therapy that can decrease the progression of the disease, but common side effects include GI disturbance and stomatitis. Dimercaprol can enhance excretion of Gold Salts if severe side effects occur.
In extreme cases, surgical procedures and joint replacement may be necessary.

Que: In managing Rheumatoid Arthritis, which habit(s) of a patient are needed for effective management?
Options:

A) Smoking cessation

B) Regular exercise

C) Consuming high-sugar foods

D) Avoiding NSAIDs altogether

E) Excessive alcohol consumption

F) Taking steroids without prescription

G) Refusing all surgical procedures

H) Increasing the intake of Gold Salts

Correct Answers: A) Smoking cessation and B) Regular exercise.

Explanation:

A) Smoking cessation: This is an important habit for effective management of Rheumatoid Arthritis. Smoking is a known risk factor for the development and progression of the disease. Quitting smoking can help improve symptoms and slow the progression of the condition.

B) Regular exercise: Regular exercise is essential for managing Rheumatoid Arthritis. It helps improve joint mobility, reduce pain, and maintain overall physical health. Exercise can also help prevent muscle atrophy and maintain joint function.

C) Consuming high-sugar foods: This is not a recommended habit for managing Rheumatoid Arthritis. High-sugar foods may contribute to inflammation and can negatively impact overall health.

D) Avoiding NSAIDs altogether: NSAIDs (non-steroidal anti-inflammatory drugs) are commonly used to reduce pain and inflammation in Rheumatoid Arthritis. Avoiding them altogether without medical guidance may not be a suitable approach to managing the condition.

E) Excessive alcohol consumption: Excessive alcohol consumption can have negative effects on overall health and may not be beneficial for managing Rheumatoid Arthritis.

F) Taking steroids without prescription: Taking steroids without a prescription and medical supervision can lead to serious side effects, including hyperglycemia. It is not a recommended habit for managing the condition.

G) Refusing all surgical procedures: In extreme cases, surgical procedures and joint replacement may be necessary for managing Rheumatoid Arthritis. Refusing all surgical procedures may not be advisable when the condition requires it.

H) Increasing the intake of Gold Salts: Increasing the intake of Gold Salts without medical guidance can lead to side effects and complications. It should be done under the supervision of a healthcare professional if deemed necessary for treatment.

Renal and Urinary System

Practice Session

Match the following lab values with their normal range:

Que : Blood urea nitrogen (BUN) level B. Serum creatinine level C. Serum sodium level D. Serum potassium level
1. 136-145 mEq/L
2. 0.7-1.3 mg/dL
3. 3.5-5.0 mEq/L
4. 6-24 mg/dL

Explanation: Blood urea nitrogen (BUN) level indicates the amount of nitrogen in the blood that comes from urea, a waste product of protein metabolism. The normal range for BUN is 6-24 mg/dL. Serum creatinine level indicates the amount of creatinine in the blood, which is a waste product produced by muscles. The normal range for serum creatinine level is 0.7-1.3 mg/dL (62-115 µmol/L). Serum sodium level measures the concentration of sodium ions in the blood. The normal range for serum sodium level is 136-145 mEq/L. Serum potassium level measures the concentration of potassium ions in the blood. The normal range for serum potassium level is 3.5-5.0 mEq/L.
Incorrect matches: Option 1 - The normal range of serum sodium level is 136-145 mEq/L, not for BUN level. Option 2 - The normal range of serum creatinine level is 0.7-1.3 mg/dL (62-115 µmol/L), not for serum potassium level. Option 4 - The normal range of serum potassium level is 3.5-5.0 mEq/L, not for BUN level.

Que : A patient who fell from a cliff has been ordered a urinary catheter insertion by the healthcare provider in the emergency department. However, the nurse preparing for the procedure observes blood at the urinary meatus.
What should the nurse do next?

1. Use a small-sized catheter.
2. Notify the healthcare provider before performing the procedure.
3. Use parenteral analgesic before the procedure.
4. Clean the meatus with soap and water before inserting the catheter.
5. Proceed with the catheterization regardless of the bleeding.
6. Apply pressure to the meatus to stop the bleeding.
7. Administer antibiotics to prevent infection.

Correct answer: 2 and 4.

Explanation: Blood at the urinary meatus is a sign of urethral trauma or disruption. It is important for the nurse to notify the healthcare provider before performing the procedure to rule out the cause of bleeding. Diagnostic testing may be required to assess the extent of injury. Cleaning the meatus with soap and water before inserting the catheter helps prevent infection. Using a smaller sized catheter (Option 1) may aggravate the injury and cause more bleeding. Parenteral analgesic (Option 3) may not be necessary if the procedure is delayed. Proceeding with the catheterization regardless of the bleeding (Option 5) can cause more damage and increase the risk of infection. Applying pressure to the meatus (Option 6) may temporarily stop the bleeding, but it does not address the underlying issue. Administering antibiotics (Option 7) is not necessary at this point since there is no confirmed infection.

Obstetrics and Gynaecology

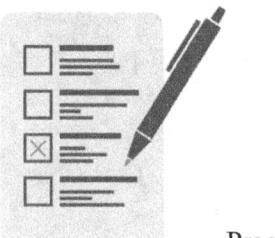

Practice Session

Reproductive System

Que : A woman has just had a radiation implant inserted into her cervix to treat her cervical cancer.

Which of the following is the appropriate care for a client with radiation implants?

A) Keep the client in a shared room

B) Permit pregnant caretakers or pregnant visitors into the room

C) Do not wear a dosimeter when providing care to clients with radiation implants

D) Keep a lead-lined container in the room for disposal of the implant should it become dislodged

E) Client should remain active and mobile

F) Use latex gloves when handling potentially contaminated secretions

Answer Explanation:

B) Permit pregnant caretakers or pregnant visitors into the room - This is incorrect as pregnant individuals should not be permitted into the room of a client with radiation implants. Pregnant individuals are at a higher risk of harm from radiation exposure, and thus should be kept away from the client.

D) Keep a lead-lined container in the room for disposal of the implant should it become dislodged - This is one of the appropriate measures for a client with radiation implants. A lead-lined container should be kept in the room to ensure safe disposal of the implant should it become dislodged.

A) Keep the client in a shared room - This is incorrect as the client should be assigned to a private room with a "Caution: Radioactive Material" sign on the door to ensure that others are aware of the potential risks.

C) Do not wear a dosimeter when providing care to clients with radiation implants - This is incorrect as all staff members providing care should wear a dosimeter during every client contact to monitor radiation exposure.

E) Client should remain active and mobile - This is incorrect as the client should remain in bed with as little movement as possible to minimize the potential dislodgment of the implant.

F) Use latex gloves when handling potentially contaminated secretions - This is one of the appropriate measures for a client with radiation implants. Latex gloves should be used when handling potentially contaminated secretions as all client secretions have the potential of being radioactive.

Que : Dr. Ranjan is a pediatrician who is conducting a neonatal assessment of a newborn baby. As part of the assessment, Dr. Ranjan checks for various physical and reflex characteristics. During the examination, Dr. Ranjan notices that the baby is lacking _____ on the entire sole of the feet. What could be the potential implications of this observation?

What physical characteristic is typically absent in premature or genetically disordered newborns?
A) Babinski reflex
B) Epstein's pearl
C) Lanugo hair
D) Planter creases

Answer: D) Planter creases.
Explanation: As mentioned, planter creases are present on the entire sole of a newborn, and their absence may indicate prematurity or a genetic disorder. Therefore, the correct answer is option D. Babinski reflex, Epstein's pearl, and lanugo hair are all physical characteristics that may be present in newborns, but their presence or absence does not necessarily indicate prematurity or a genetic disorder.

A) Babinski reflex: The Babinski reflex is a primitive reflex that is present in newborns. It is elicited by stroking the lateral surface of the sole of the foot, which causes the toes to hyperextend and fan out. This reflex is normally present in newborns and typically disappears around 12 months of age. The presence or absence of the Babinski reflex can be an indicator of neurologic health in a newborn. In some cases, the Babinski reflex may persist beyond infancy, which can be a sign of a neurologic disorder.

B) Epstein's pearl: Epstein's pearl is a white, pearl-like epithelial cyst that can appear on the gums or palate of newborns. These cysts are harmless and typically disappear within a few weeks after birth. Epstein's pearls are caused by trapped epithelial cells during the development of the baby's mouth.

C) Lanugo hair: Lanugo hair is fine, downy hair that covers the entire body of some newborns. This hair is typically present on premature infants and usually disappears by the time the baby reaches full term. Lanugo hair is thought to help regulate the baby's body temperature and protect their skin in utero.

D) Planter creases: Planter creases are the lines or creases that appear on the entire sole of the feet of newborns. These creases are formed during fetal development and are present in most newborns. The absence of planter creases on the entire sole of the feet may indicate prematurity or a genetic disorder, such as Down syndrome. However, the absence of planter creases alone is not enough to diagnose a disorder and further evaluation and testing would be needed to confirm any potential issues.

Que : A 32-year-old pregnant patient was admitted to the labor and delivery unit for induction of labor due to medical reasons. The medical team decided to use oxytocin to facilitate labor progress. The oxytocin infusion was started at a low dose and gradually increased based on the patient's response.. After some time, the medical team immediately stopped the oxytocin infusion and performed an emergency cesarean birth to deliver the baby safely.

What potential risks can oxytocin use carry during labor induction or augmentation in pregnant patients?

A) Increase the risk of placenta previa during pregnancy.
B) Delay milk production in the postpartum period.
C) Cause contractions that are too strong or frequent, leading to reduced placental blood flow and non-assuring fetal heart patterns.
D) Increase the risk of postpartum hemorrhage.

Explanation: Option A is incorrect because oxytocin does not increase the risk of placenta previa during pregnancy. Option B is incorrect because oxytocin does not delay milk production in the postpartum period. In fact, oxytocin can decrease postpartum hemorrhage by promoting uterine contractions after birth. Option C is the correct answer because oxytocin can cause contractions that are too strong or frequent, leading to reduced placental blood flow and non-assuring fetal heart patterns, such as late deceleration, fetal bradycardia, tachycardia, or minimal variability, which may require emergency cesarean birth. It is important for medical professionals to carefully monitor the use of oxytocin during labor induction or augmentation to prevent potential risks to the mother and baby. Option D is incorrect because oxytocin can actually decrease the risk of postpartum hemorrhage by promoting uterine contractions after birth.

Que : Mrs. Malla gave birth to a healthy baby girl at 8:00 AM. The nurse on duty is now monitoring her during the third stage of labor or the active phase. Which of the following is not a sign of placental separation during the active phase?

A. Lengthening of umbilical cord
B. Sudden gush of vaginal blood
C. Change in the shape of uterus (globular in shape)
D. Appearance of placenta in vaginal opening

Answer: D. Appearance of placenta in vaginal opening

Explanation: During the active phase or third stage of labor, placental separation occurs. The signs of placental separation include lengthening of the umbilical cord, sudden gush of vaginal blood, change in the shape of the uterus (globular in shape), and firm uterine contractions. The appearance of the placenta in the vaginal opening is a sign of placental expulsion, which is the second phase of the third stage of labor. Placental expulsion occurs after placental separation and is characterized by the expulsion of the placenta using gentle traction on the cord. Therefore, option D is incorrect.

During the active phase or third stage of labor, it is essential for nurses to provide appropriate nursing care to the mother to prevent complications such as infection and hemorrhage. The nursing care tips during the active phase include coaching the mother in relaxation for the delivery of the placenta, congratulating her on the delivery of the baby, encouraging skin-to-skin contact to facilitate bonding and early breastfeeding, administering prophylactic oxytocin as ordered, utilizing controlled cord traction technique for placental expulsion, and utilizing absorbable synthetic suture materials for primary repair of episiotomy or perineal lacerations. It is also crucial for nurses to check the vital signs and monitor for excessive bleeding during the immediate postpartum period. The WHO recommendations for immediate postpartum include early resumption of feeding, prophylactic antibiotics for women who sustained third to fourth-degree perineal tear during delivery, and early postpartum discharge for healthy women who delivered vaginally to term infants. The routine use of ice packs and oral methylergometrine for patients who delivered vaginally are not recommended during immediate postpartum.

Que : A pregnant client with severe preeclampsia develops seizures. The nurse's immediate intervention should include:

A. Administering pain medication
B. Placing the client in a supine position
C. Turning the client on her side and administering oxygen by face mask
D. Administering oxytocin to induce labor

Correct answer: C. Turning the client on her side and administering oxygen by face mask

Explanation:

Preeclampsia is a pregnancy-related condition marked by elevated blood pressure and evidence of damage to organs, especially the liver and kidneys. It generally arises after the 20th week of pregnancy and can swiftly advance to eclampsia, which involves seizures, potential cerebral hemorrhage, and risks to both maternal and fetal lives. Symptoms of preeclampsia may be absent or include headaches, visual changes, nausea, and swelling. Managing preeclampsia involves rigorous monitoring of blood pressure, protein in urine, and fetal health, along with medications such as antihypertensives and magnesium sulfate to avert seizures. The only conclusive treatment for preeclampsia is the delivery of the baby and placenta, though this must be weighed against the risks associated with premature delivery.

In cases of severe preeclampsia where seizures occur, this signals the onset of eclampsia, a critical emergency needing prompt action. The nurse should stay with the patient, seek additional help, and ensure the airway remains clear by positioning the patient on her side. This posture reduces the risk of aspiration and enhances blood flow to the placenta. Oxygen should be provided via face mask at 8 to 10 L/min to maintain adequate oxygen levels for the placenta. Pain relief is not suitable since it does not address the root cause of the seizures. The supine position should be avoided to prevent compromising fetal blood flow. Inducing labor with oxytocin is not advised until the patient is stabilized and the fetus is in a safe condition. Continuous monitoring of the fetal heart rate is essential, and magnesium sulfate may be administered to prevent further seizures. Following the seizure, the nurse should insert an oral airway to ensure the airway remains open and perform suctioning as necessary. If stabilization occurs, preparations for fetal delivery should be made. Comprehensive documentation of the seizure, the patient's response, and the outcome is also crucial.

Que: A pregnant client arrives at the hospital with umbilical cord prolapse. The nurse takes immediate action to relieve cord pressure and provide appropriate care. Which of the following actions are appropriate for the nurse to take?

A. Administer pain medication to the client

B. Elevate the fetal presenting part that is lying on the cord by applying finger pressure with a gloved hand
C. Push the cord into the uterus
D. Place the client in a prone position

Answer: B

Explanation:

Umbilical cord prolapse is a critical situation where the umbilical cord slips alongside or beneath the fetus's presenting part and may be visible or palpable in the vagina. In such emergencies, the nurse must promptly alleviate the pressure on the cord to ensure sufficient oxygen supply to the fetus. To do this, gently pressing with a gloved finger to lift the presenting part off the cord is a suitable method to reduce cord compression.

Administering pain medication to the client (Option A) is not a priority in this situation, and it does not address the emergency. Pushing the cord into the uterus (Option C) is also not appropriate because it can cause cord compression and decrease blood flow to the fetus. Placing the client in a prone position (Option D) is not recommended as it may increase cord compression and worsen the condition.

Therefore, the correct answer is B.

Eyes and Ears

A 27-year-old mechanic arrives at the emergency department with a chemical burn to his right eye after an accidental splash of car battery acid.

Multiple Choice Question

Which of the following statements is true regarding the management of this chemical eye injury?

A. The eye should be irrigated with tap water for 5 minutes.

B. The pH of the eye should be measured before starting irrigation.

C. Irrigation should continue until the eye's pH is restored to the normal range of 6 to 7.

D. The patient should be positioned with the head tilted away from the affected eye during irrigation.

E. Documenting the type of chemical involved is not necessary if irrigation is effective.

Correct Answer: C. Irrigation should continue until the eye's pH is restored to the normal range of 6 to 7.

Explanation:

A. The eye should be irrigated with tap water for 5 minutes.

Wrong. Tap water is not recommended for eye irrigation as it may contain impurities; sterile saline or specific ocular irrigants should be used. Irrigation should also continue for a minimum of 10 minutes, not just 5.

B. The pH of the eye should be measured before starting irrigation.

Wrong. The pH of the eye is typically measured after irrigation to assess whether the chemical has been sufficiently neutralized.

C. Irrigation should continue until the eye's pH is restored to the normal range of 6 to 7.

Correct. It is essential to continue irrigation until the pH of the eye returns to the normal range to ensure complete neutralization of the chemical.

D. The patient should be positioned with the head tilted away from the affected eye during irrigation.

Wrong. The patient should be positioned with the head tilted toward the affected side to facilitate effective drainage of the chemical out of the eye.

E. Documenting the type of chemical involved is not necessary if irrigation is effective.

Wrong. Identifying and documenting the type of chemical is crucial for determining appropriate treatment and follow-up care, even if the irrigation is effective.

Que: Which statement is correct regarding activities to avoid after cataract surgery?

A. You should engage in heavy lifting as long as the weight is less than 10 lbs (4.5 kg).

B. It is safe to rub your eyes gently to relieve itching after surgery.

C. It is important to avoid sudden movements and lifting objects heavier than 5 lbs (2.25 kg).

D. You can perform strenuous activities like running without any restrictions.

E. Sneezing and coughing are fine as long as they are not accompanied by other activities.

Correct Answer: C. It is important to avoid sudden movements and lifting objects heavier than 5 lbs (2.25 kg).

Explanation:

A. You should engage in heavy lifting as long as the weight is less than 10 lbs (4.5 kg).

Incorrect. Lifting any weight heavier than 5 lbs (2.25 kg) is advised against to prevent strain on the eye, regardless of the weight.

B. It is safe to rub your eyes gently to relieve itching after surgery.

Incorrect. Rubbing your eyes can cause harm and should be avoided to protect the surgical site and promote healing.

C. It is important to avoid sudden movements and lifting objects heavier than 5 lbs (2.25 kg).

Correct. Avoiding sudden movements and heavy lifting is crucial to prevent strain and potential complications during recovery.

D. You can perform strenuous activities like running without any restrictions.

Incorrect. Strenuous activities should be avoided as they can put undue stress on the healing eye.

E. Sneezing and coughing are fine as long as they are not accompanied by other activities.

Incorrect. Sneezing and coughing should be minimized as they can cause strain and potentially disrupt the healing process.

Que: Which statement is correct about the management of Primary Angle-Closure Glaucoma (PACG)?

A) PACG requires ongoing medication to manage chronic symptoms.

B) Emergency treatment for PACG involves medications to lower intraocular pressure (IOP) and potential surgical intervention.

C) Primary Open-Angle Glaucoma (POAG) is treated with surgery to correct the angle of the eye.

D) PACG typically causes a gradual, painless loss of peripheral vision over time.

Correct Answer: B) Emergency treatment for PACG involves medications to lower intraocular pressure (IOP) and potential surgical intervention.

Explanation:

A) Incorrect. PACG requires emergency treatment rather than ongoing chronic management; medications to lower IOP are administered urgently, and surgery may be necessary.

B) Correct. PACG is an emergency condition that requires prompt treatment to lower IOP and might involve surgical intervention.

C) Incorrect. POAG is treated with medications to lower IOP, not surgery to correct the angle of the eye. PACG involves issues with the angle.

D) Incorrect. PACG causes sudden symptoms including blurred vision and halos around lights, not gradual and painless loss of peripheral vision.

Which statement is accurate regarding cochlear implants?

A) Cochlear implants are primarily used for conductive hearing loss.

B) Cochlear implants use a small computer to convert electrical signals into sound waves.

C) Electrodes from cochlear implants are placed outside the ear canal.

D) Cochlear implants stimulate auditory nerve fibers directly with electrical impulses.

E) Cochlear implants amplify sound to make it louder, not clearer.

Correct Answer: D) Cochlear implants stimulate auditory nerve fibers directly with electrical impulses.

Explanation:

A) Incorrect. Cochlear implants are designed to address sensorineural hearing loss, not conductive hearing loss.

B) Incorrect. Cochlear implants convert sound waves into electrical signals, not the other way around.

C) Incorrect. Electrodes for cochlear implants are positioned inside the ear, not outside.

D) Correct. Cochlear implants work by directly stimulating auditory nerve fibers with electrical impulses.

E) Incorrect. Cochlear implants do not simply amplify sound; they transform sound into electrical signals to stimulate the auditory nerve.

Case Study: Mr. Thompson recently received a hearing aid. To ensure its proper functioning and longevity, he followed all the recommended guidelines for usage and care.

What is the best practice to prevent feedback noise when using a hearing aid?

A) Increase the volume to the highest level.

B) Store the hearing aid in a damp environment.

C) Clean the ear mold with any household cleaner.

D) Turn off the hearing aid before removing it from the ear and remove the battery when not in use.

E) Use hairspray around the hearing aid to maintain its appearance.

Correct Answer: D) Turn off the hearing aid before removing it from the ear and remove the battery when not in use.

Explanation:

A) Incorrect. Increasing the volume can actually increase feedback noise, not prevent it.

B) Incorrect. Storing the hearing aid in a damp environment can damage it, not prevent feedback.

C) Incorrect. Using household cleaners can damage the hearing aid; it should be cleaned according to the manufacturer's instructions.

D) Correct. Turning off the hearing aid before removal and removing the battery helps prevent feedback and prolongs the device's life.

E) Incorrect. Hairspray and other products can harm the hearing aid's receiver and should be kept away from it.

Which of the following medications is known to potentially cause hearing loss?

A. Ibuprofen

B. Ethacrynic acid

C. Vancomycin

D. Chloramphenicol

Correct Answer: B. Ethacrynic acid and C. Vancomycin

Explanation:

A. Ibuprofen

Explanation: Ibuprofen is a nonsteroidal anti-inflammatory drug (NSAID) commonly used for pain relief and inflammation. While it can have side effects, it is generally not associated with hearing loss when used at recommended doses. High doses or prolonged use can potentially lead to tinnitus or other ear-related symptoms, but this is rare.

B. Ethacrynic acid

Explanation: Ethacrynic acid is a diuretic that can affect hearing. It is known to cause ototoxicity, which can lead to hearing loss. This risk is particularly relevant in higher doses or prolonged use. Ototoxicity in diuretics like ethacrynic acid occurs due to the drug's effect on the inner ear's fluid balance.

C. Vancomycin

Explanation: Vancomycin is an antibiotic used to treat serious bacterial infections. It can potentially cause hearing loss, especially if used in high doses or if the patient has pre-existing kidney issues.

D. Chloramphenicol

Explanation: Chloramphenicol is an antibiotic known for its potential to cause aplastic anemia, but it is not commonly associated with hearing loss. Hearing loss related to antibiotics is more commonly associated with aminoglycosides, such as gentamicin or streptomycin, rather than chloramphenicol.

Que: Which of the following side effects is commonly associated with glaucoma medications?

A. Nausea

B. Myopia

C. Drowsiness

D. Rash

Correct Answer: B. Myopia

Explanation:

A. Nausea: This is not a common side effect of glaucoma medications. Some medications may have gastrointestinal side effects, but nausea is not prevalent.

B. Myopia: Glaucoma medications, particularly those affecting the pupil and ciliary muscle, can lead to changes in vision, including myopia.

C. Drowsiness: While some medications may cause drowsiness, it is not a typical side effect of glaucoma medications.

D. Rash: A rash is not commonly associated with glaucoma medications and is more likely related to allergic reactions or other types of medication.

Cardiovascular System/circulatory disorders

Practice Session

Que: Which of the following diagnostic studies is most useful in providing a definitive diagnosis of angina?

A. Electrocardiography

B. Stress testing

C. Cardiac enzyme and troponin levels

D. Cardiac catheterization

E. Magnetic resonance imaging

Correct answers: D

Explanation:

Cardiac catheterization (Option D) is the most useful diagnostic study in providing a definitive diagnosis of angina as it provides information about the patency of the coronary arteries. This test involves inserting a catheter into the heart and injecting contrast dye to visualize the coronary arteries.

Electrocardiography (Option A) can provide important information about the heart's electrical activity during an episode of pain, but it is not a definitive diagnostic tool for angina.

Stress testing (Option B) can also provide information about the presence of myocardial ischemia, but it is not as definitive as cardiac catheterization.

Cardiac enzyme and troponin levels (Option C) are useful in diagnosing myocardial infarction but are not diagnostic for angina.

Magnetic resonance imaging (Option E) can provide detailed images of the heart and blood vessels but is not routinely used in the diagnosis of angina.

Que : A patient with a history of heart attack is on warfarin drug therapy. Which of the following can be advised to the patient ?

1. Proper oral care by brushing with soft brushes and hygiene should be followed.
2. Change your diet to nutritious green leafy vegetables such as spinach, cabbage, broccoli, collard greens, lettuce etc.
3. Alcoholic beverages can be taken occassionally only.
4. Side effects such as blood in the stool and urine are normal for drugs in this class.

Answer:

The correct answer to this Que is option 1. The drug may cause bleeding from the gums. Proper oral hygiene and brushing with soft bristle brushes should be done.

Option 2 is incorrect. Changes in diet or use of other drugs can alter their risk of bleeding and/or clotting. sudden change in diet such as spinach, cabbage, broccoli, collard greens, lettuce which contains vitamin k should be avoided.
Option 3 is incorrect. The patient shouldn't take any alcoholic beverages as it interferes with the drug.
Option 4 is incorrect. A black box warning is the FDA's most stringent warning for drugs and medical devices on the market. Warfarin can cause major or fatal bleeding. So whenever, you see such conditions the health care worker must be informed.

Que : A client is complaining of dizziness and has shortness of breath. She shows heart rate of 42 beats per minute and upon reading, the BP it is clear than hypotension with a reading of 85/55. Which of the following could be the causes of this problem ?

i. Her blood glucose level of 100

ii. She is prescribed atropine

iii. She could be suffering from some viral ever.

iv. She is prescribed digoxin

The correct answer to this Que is the last option that is 'She is prescribed with digoxin'. We learnt that certain drugs such as digoxin cause bradycardia and these all symptoms that she is showing such as dizziness, shortness of breath and hypotension are the symptoms of bradycardia.

Que : Which of the following EKG strip shows the atrial fibrillation ?

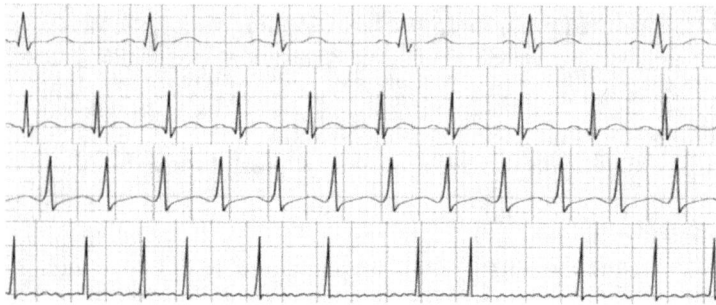

Answer:

The first strip is for normal sinus.

The second for sinus tachycardia.

The third is for supraventricular tachycardia and the correct answer is the last option.

Normal Sinus Rhythm (NSR) is characterized by an upright and smooth P wave, indicating normal atrial depolarization. The PR interval ranges between 120 and 200 milliseconds, reflecting normal conduction through the AV node. The QRS complex is narrow, less than 120 milliseconds, showing that ventricular depolarization is normal. The T wave is upright, following the QRS complex, and the heart rate typically falls between 60 and 100 beats per minute.

Sinus Tachycardia maintains an upright P wave similar to that seen in NSR. The PR interval remains within the normal range, and the QRS complex is still narrow. The T wave is also upright. However, the heart rate exceeds 100 beats per minute, indicating a faster rhythm while still preserving a regular pattern and normal P wave morphology.

Supraventricular Tachycardia (SVT) often features absent or merged P waves that can be difficult to identify due to the rapid rate. The PR interval is hard to measure accurately, and the QRS complex remains narrow. The T wave is often indistinct because of the rapid heart rate. The heart rate usually exceeds 150 beats per minute and presents a regular rhythm, although the individual waves can be challenging to discern.

Atrial Fibrillation (AF) is marked by the absence of distinct P waves, replaced instead by irregular, fibrillatory waves. The PR interval is not applicable due to the lack of P waves. The QRS complex is narrow, but the T wave is irregular. The heart rate in AF is typically irregularly rapid, reflecting the erratic nature of the rhythm.

You can see that the strip for supraventricular tachycardia and atrial fibrillation is lot similar but still you can identify it with supraventricular tachycardia as atrial fibrillation is very unrythmic. We know that supraventricular tachycardia has normal rhythm and supraventricular tachycardia shows frequent QRS complex. So, you won't see much any other waves in between these QRS complex in supraventricular tachycardia.

Gastrointestinal disorders

Practice Session

Que : Ms. Alvin, a 60-year-old female with a history of hypertension, presents to the clinic with complaints of heartburn and acid reflux. Upon examination, the provider prescribes an antacid for her symptoms.

Aluminum compounds can cause _____ while reducing the effects of tetracyclines, warfarin sodium, and digoxin.

A) Hypertension
B) Hypophosphatemia
C) Hypernatremia
D) Constipation
E) Acid rebound
F) Diarrhea

Answer: B) Hypophosphatemia and D) Constipation

Explanation: Aluminum hydroxide is used to treat hyperphosphatemia, but it can also cause hypophosphatemia by reducing phosphate absorption. This medication should be used with caution in patients with renal impairment. Options A and C are incorrect because aluminum compounds do not contain significant amounts of sodium nor do they cause hypertension. Option D is a common side effect of aluminum compounds. Option E is a side effect of calcium compounds, not aluminum compounds. Option F is a side effect of magnesium compounds.

Que : A 35-year-old female patient presents to the healthcare facility with complaints of abdominal pain and diarrhea. She was diagnosed with Crohn's disease in the past. On assessment, she reports fever, crampy and colicky pain after meals, diarrhea (semisolid) with mucus and pus, abdominal distention, anorexia, nausea, vomiting, weight loss, anemia, dehydration, electrolyte imbalances, and malnutrition. Which of the following interventions should the nurse prioritize for this patient?

Which of the following interventions should the nurse prioritize for the patient with Crohn's disease?
A. Encourage a low-fiber diet
B. Administer high-dose corticosteroids
C. Provide parenteral nutrition
D. Administer antidiarrheal medication
E. Avoid surgery as long as possible
F. Administer antibiotics

Correct Answers: C, E

Explanation: The nurse should prioritize providing parenteral nutrition (Option C) and avoiding surgery as long as possible (Option E) for the patient with Crohn's disease. This disease can lead to malnutrition due to malabsorption of nutrients, and it is important to provide adequate nutrition to the patient. Surgery is avoided for as long as possible because recurrence of the disease process in the same region is likely to occur. Low-fiber diet (Option A) is not recommended for Crohn's disease as it can aggravate the condition. High-dose corticosteroids (Option B) may be used for acute exacerbations, but it is not the priority intervention in this case. Antidiarrheal medication (Option D) is not recommended for Crohn's disease as it can worsen the condition. Antibiotics (Option F) may be used to treat bacterial infections in patients with Crohn's disease but it is not the priority intervention in this case.

Note: It is important to provide education to the patient about their condition and how to manage it. The nurse should encourage the patient to follow a high-protein, high-calorie diet and drink plenty of fluids. The nurse should also monitor the patient's electrolyte levels and administer electrolyte replacement therapy as necessary.

Que : Saigrace is a 34-year-old man who is admitted to the hospital with a diagnosis of ulcerative colitis. His medical history includes asthma and seasonal allergies. He has a history of smoking, but has quit for the past year.

Which of the following is a characteristic of ulcerative colitis?

A) It results in excessive absorption of nutrients
B) It begins in the cecum and spreads downwards
C) It causes loss of elasticity and inability to absorb nutrients
D) It is not characterized by periods of remissions and exacerbations

Answer: C) It causes loss of elasticity and inability to absorb nutrients

Explanation: Ulcerative colitis is an inflammatory disease that affects the colon and rectum. It causes inflammation, ulcers, and bleeding in the colon, leading to the development of scar tissue, which can result in a loss of elasticity and the ability to absorb nutrients. Option A is incorrect because ulcerative colitis results in poor absorption of nutrients, not excessive absorption. Option B is incorrect because ulcerative colitis commonly begins in the rectum and spreads upward toward the cecum, not the other way around. Option D is incorrect because ulcerative colitis is characterized by various periods of remissions and exacerbations.

PART II: PHARMACOLOGICAL INTERVENTIONS

Antibiotics: Introduction and classification

Penicillin: Used to treat a variety of bacterial infections such as strep throat, ear infections, and pneumonia. Nursing considerations include assessing for penicillin allergies, monitoring for adverse reactions such as anaphylaxis, and advising patients to take the medication as prescribed.

Amoxicillin: A broad-spectrum antibiotic effective against many bacterial infections, including sinusitis, bronchitis, and urinary tract infections. Nurses should monitor for allergic reactions, educate patients about completing the full course, and advise on potential side effects like diarrhea.

Cephalexin: Often prescribed for skin infections, urinary tract infections, and respiratory tract infections. Nursing considerations involve monitoring for allergic reactions, educating patients on proper administration, and advising on potential interactions with other medications.

Ciprofloxacin: Used to treat urinary tract infections, respiratory tract infections, and certain types of bacterial diarrhea. Nurses need to monitor for adverse reactions like tendon rupture, educate patients to avoid sun exposure, and advise against taking with dairy products or antacids.

Azithromycin: Effective against respiratory tract infections, skin infections, and sexually transmitted diseases like chlamydia. Nursing management includes assessing for allergies, educating patients about potential GI upset, and advising on the importance of completing the full course.

Doxycycline: Treats a wide range of infections, including acne, respiratory tract infections, and sexually transmitted diseases like gonorrhea. Nurses should monitor for photosensitivity reactions, advise patients to take with food to minimize GI upset, and educate about the risk of vaginal yeast infections.

Metronidazole: Used to treat infections caused by certain types of bacteria and parasites, including bacterial vaginosis and certain types of anaerobic infections. Nursing considerations include monitoring for side effects like metallic taste and advising patients to avoid alcohol consumption.

Sulfamethoxazole/Trimethoprim: Effective against urinary tract infections, respiratory tract infections, and certain types of bacterial diarrhea. Nurses should monitor for allergic reactions, educate patients about potential side effects like rash or nausea, and advise on the importance of staying hydrated.

Levofloxacin: Treats a variety of bacterial infections, including respiratory tract infections and urinary tract infections. Nursing management involves monitoring for tendonitis or tendon rupture, educating patients about potential side effects like dizziness, and advising against taking with dairy products or antacids.

Erythromycin: Used to treat respiratory tract infections, skin infections, and certain sexually transmitted diseases like syphilis. Nurses should monitor for allergic reactions, educate patients about potential GI upset, and advise on the importance of taking the medication on an empty stomach.

Practice Session

Que: Anita is a 28-year-old female with a history of recurrent urinary tract infections (UTIs). She presents to the clinic with symptoms of dysuria, urinary frequency, and suprapubic discomfort. Anita's medical history includes a penicillin allergy, and she is currently taking warfarin for a previous deep vein thrombosis (DVT).

The provider suspects a UTI and orders a urine culture. Pending culture results, the provider wants to initiate empirical antibiotic therapy to alleviate Anita's symptoms.

Which antibiotic(s) would be the most appropriate choice for empirical therapy in Anita's case, considering her penicillin allergy and concurrent warfarin therapy?

A. Cephalexin

B. Azithromycin

C. Nitrofurantoin

D. Ciprofloxacin

E. Amoxicillin-Clavulanate

F. Trimethoprim/Sulfamethoxazole

G. Clindamycin

Explanation:

A. Cephalexin

Wrong: Although cephalexin is a cephalosporin and not a penicillin, there is a potential for cross-reactivity in patients with penicillin allergies. Additionally, cephalexin can interact with warfarin, increasing the risk of bleeding.

B. Azithromycin

Wrong: Azithromycin is not typically used for UTIs as it is more effective against respiratory infections and certain sexually transmitted infections. It also has potential interactions with warfarin, which could increase the risk of bleeding.

C. Nitrofurantoin

Right: Nitrofurantoin is a good choice for uncomplicated UTIs and is generally safe for patients with penicillin allergies. It has minimal interaction with warfarin, making it a safer option for Anita.

D. Ciprofloxacin

Wrong: While ciprofloxacin is effective for UTIs, it has significant interactions with warfarin, increasing the risk of bleeding. It is also associated with potential side effects like tendonitis and tendon rupture.

E. Amoxicillin-Clavulanate

Wrong: Amoxicillin-Clavulanate is a penicillin derivative and should be avoided in patients with penicillin allergies.

F. Trimethoprim/Sulfamethoxazole

Wrong: Although effective for UTIs, Trimethoprim/Sulfamethoxazole can interact with warfarin, increasing the risk of bleeding. Additionally, there is a risk of sulfa allergy, which needs to be considered.

G. Clindamycin

Wrong: Clindamycin is not typically used for UTIs as it is more effective against anaerobic infections. It also has potential interactions with warfarin, increasing the risk of bleeding.

Que: A 25-year-old patient taking tetracycline for acne reports experiencing nausea, sensitivity to sunlight, and notices their teeth becoming discolored.

Which of the following adverse effects is **least likely** associated with tetracyclines?

A) Gastrointestinal discomfort
B) Teeth discoloration
C) Photosensitivity
D) Hepatotoxicity
E) Ototoxicity

Correct Answer: E) Ototoxicity

Explanation of Each Option

A) Gastrointestinal discomfort

- **Why it's wrong:** Gastrointestinal issues, like nausea or vomiting, are common side effects of tetracyclines. The patient's report of nausea aligns with typical gastrointestinal effects of this medication.

B) Teeth discoloration

- **Why it's wrong:** Tetracyclines can cause teeth staining, especially in children or young adults, as their teeth are still developing. This adverse effect is well-documented for this drug class.

C) Photosensitivity

- **Why it's wrong:** Photosensitivity is a common adverse reaction seen with tetracycline use, making the patient more susceptible to sunburns and skin rashes, which aligns with the patient's experience.

D) Hepatotoxicity

- **Why it's wrong:** Hepatotoxicity, although less frequent, can occur with tetracyclines, especially at higher doses. Liver toxicity is a known, though relatively uncommon, side effect of this drug class.

E) Ototoxicity

- **Why it's right:** Tetracyclines are not commonly associated with ototoxicity (hearing issues). This is more characteristic of other medications like aminoglycosides, making it the least likely adverse effect linked to tetracyclines in this scenario.

A 40-year-old patient on an aminoglycoside antibiotic for a bacterial infection reports experiencing ringing in the ears, dizziness, and a decrease in urine output.

Que: Which of the following patient statements indicates an adverse effect **least likely** associated with aminoglycosides?

A) "I have been experiencing ringing in my ears."
B) "I've felt dizzy and off-balance lately."
C) "I noticed a significant decrease in my urine output."
D) "I have sensitivity to sunlight."
E) "My hearing seems to have gotten worse."

Correct Answer: D) "I have sensitivity to sunlight."

Explanation of Each Option

A) "I have been experiencing ringing in my ears."

- **Why it's wrong:** Tinnitus, or ringing in the ears, is a common symptom of ototoxicity, which is a well-known adverse effect of aminoglycosides. This aligns with the reported side effects of the drug.

B) "I've felt dizzy and off-balance lately."

- **Why it's wrong:** Dizziness and balance issues can occur as part of the vestibular toxicity associated with aminoglycosides, which affects the inner ear.

C) "I noticed a significant decrease in my urine output."

- **Why it's wrong:** Aminoglycosides are known to cause nephrotoxicity, which can manifest as reduced urine output, making this statement a plausible adverse effect.

D) "I have sensitivity to sunlight."

- **Why it's right:** Photosensitivity is not a typical adverse effect of aminoglycosides. This is more commonly associated with drugs like tetracyclines, making this statement the least likely adverse effect.

E) "My hearing seems to have gotten worse."

- **Why it's wrong:** Aminoglycosides are well known for causing ototoxicity, which can lead to hearing loss. Therefore, worsening hearing is a plausible adverse effect of this medication.

A nurse is assessing a patient who has been on a course of fluoroquinolone antibiotics for a bacterial infection. The patient reports experiencing muscle pain, mood changes, and light sensitivity.

Que: Which of the following nurse's statements indicates a potential adverse effect **least likely** linked to fluoroquinolone antibiotics?

A) "The muscle pain you're experiencing might be related to tendon issues caused by this antibiotic."
B) "Light sensitivity is a common reaction, so use sunscreen when going outside."
C) "Mood changes can sometimes happen as a side effect of this medication."
D) "Hearing issues are likely linked to this antibiotic treatment."
E) "Tendon problems, including tendonitis or even rupture, can occur with this medication."

Correct Answer: D) "Hearing issues are likely linked to this antibiotic treatment."

Explanation of Each Option

A) "The muscle pain you're experiencing might be related to tendon issues caused by this antibiotic."

- **Why it's wrong:** Fluoroquinolones are associated with tendonitis and tendon rupture, which can present as muscle or tendon pain. This is a typical adverse effect of this class of antibiotics.

B) "Light sensitivity is a common reaction, so use sunscreen when going outside."

- **Why it's wrong:** Photosensitivity is a known adverse effect of fluoroquinolones, so advising the patient to use sunscreen is appropriate.

C) "Mood changes can sometimes happen as a side effect of this medication."

- **Why it's wrong:** Mood changes, such as anxiety or depression, can occur with fluoroquinolone use, especially in susceptible patients.

D) "Hearing issues are likely linked to this antibiotic treatment."

- **Why it's right:** Hearing problems are not typically associated with fluoroquinolones. Hearing loss is more commonly linked to aminoglycosides, making this statement the least relevant to fluoroquinolones.

E) "Tendon problems, including tendonitis or even rupture, can occur with this medication."

- **Why it's wrong:** Tendonitis and tendon rupture are significant adverse effects of fluoroquinolones, making this statement accurate for this antibiotic.

NSAIDS AND OPOIDS: Introduction and classification

Understanding NSAIDs is crucial for NCLEX exam preparation, as they are commonly used for pain relief, inflammation reduction, and fever reduction. NSAIDs can be classified into traditional NSAIDs like ibuprofen, COX-2 inhibitors such as celecoxib, and aspirin (ASA), each with distinct mechanisms of action. While NSAIDs possess antipyretic and anti-inflammatory properties, they also pose risks such as peptic ulcers, platelet inhibition, prolonged bleeding time, and pregnancy concerns. Drug interactions, known as the "Three A's," involve interactions with anticoagulants, antihypertensives, and other NSAIDs, increasing bleeding and gastrointestinal issues. Strategies for NCLEX exam readiness include mastering pharmacology fundamentals, differentiating between NSAIDs and opioids, and assessing patient-specific factors for safe medication administration. Nurses should prioritize patient education, advocate for alternative pain management when necessary, and recognize signs of opioid overdose for prompt intervention, ensuring patient-centered care and optimal therapeutic outcomes.

Practice Session

Jane, a 45-year-old woman, presents to the emergency department with severe abdominal pain. She has a history of peptic ulcer disease and is currently taking prescribed medications for it. Jane's pain is rated 8/10 on the pain scale, and the healthcare provider orders pain management. The provider considers administering either an NSAID or an opioid for pain relief.

Select which of the statements given by the patient indicates a need for further assessment and consideration before deciding on the pain management option:

A. Jane reports a history of peptic ulcer disease.

B. Jane's pain is rated 8/10 on the pain scale.

C. Jane is currently taking medications for her peptic ulcer.

D. Jane has previously taken ibuprofen for headaches without any issues.

E. Jane mentions that she has allergies to seafood.

F. Jane has been experiencing this pain for the past 24 hours.

G. Jane states that she is currently breastfeeding her newborn.

Explanation:

The correct options are A, C, and G.

A. Jane reports a history of peptic ulcer disease: This statement is crucial for assessment because NSAIDs can exacerbate gastric ulcers. Therefore, the patient's history of peptic ulcer disease requires consideration before choosing a pain management option. This statement is correct.

C. Jane is currently taking medications for her peptic ulcer: This statement is also significant as it indicates an ongoing medical condition. The choice of pain management should be made with consideration of her current medications and potential interactions. This statement is correct.

G. Jane states that she is currently breastfeeding her newborn: This statement is important because medications can pass into breast milk and affect the infant. It is essential to consider the safety of pain management options for a breastfeeding mother. This statement is correct.

Now, let's analyze the incorrect options:

B. Jane's pain is rated 8/10 on the pain scale: While pain intensity is relevant, it does not provide information about the choice between NSAIDs and opioids specifically in the context of her medical history and current medications. This statement is not directly related to the choice of pain management in her case.

D. Jane has previously taken ibuprofen for headaches without any issues: This statement, while informative, does not address the current situation and does not provide guidance on choosing between NSAIDs and opioids in a patient with a history of peptic ulcer disease. It is not directly related to the assessment of the current pain management options.

E. Jane mentions that she has allergies to seafood: Although allergies are important to consider, this statement is not directly related to choosing between NSAIDs and opioids. It would be more relevant if the questions were about potential allergies to the selected medication.

F. Jane has been experiencing this pain for the past 24 hours: The duration of pain is relevant but does not provide specific guidance on the choice between NSAIDs and opioids in a patient with a history of peptic ulcer disease. It is not directly related to the assessment of the current pain management options.

In summary, when assessing the choice between NSAIDs and opioids for pain management in a patient with a history of peptic ulcer disease, the patient's medical history, current medications, and breastfeeding status should be carefully considered. These factors can impact the safety and efficacy of the selected pain management option.

Que: A 45-year-old patient, Mr. Johnson, presents to the pain management clinic with complaints of chronic non-cancer pain in his lower back. He has been experiencing this pain for the past five years and has tried various conservative treatments with minimal relief. As part of his pain management plan, the nurse is responsible for assessing, educating, and providing care to Mr. Johnson.

Select which of the statements given by the nurse indicates that she doesn't know the appropriate strategies for managing opioid therapy for chronic pain?

A) The nurse ensures that Mr. Johnson has a locked cabinet to store his opioids.

B) The nurse regularly assesses Mr. Johnson's pain control and watches for signs of opioid tolerance or dependence.

C) The nurse recommends an NSAID for pain management, considering Mr. Johnson's recent history of GI bleeding.

D) The nurse administers naloxone to Mr. Johnson as a preventive measure before any opioid is given.

E) The nurse recognizes that individual variations in pharmacogenetics can impact drug metabolism and adjusts the opioid dose accordingly.

F) The nurse develops a comprehensive pain management plan for Mr. Johnson, including psychological support for his history of depression.

G) The nurse escalates Mr. Johnson's opioid dose without monitoring for signs of tolerance or dependence.

H) The nurse informs Mr. Johnson that opioids can be safely stored in any accessible location within his home.

Explanation:

A) Correct: This statement indicates that the nurse is following the strategy of educating patients on safe storage of medications. It is essential to store opioids in a locked cabinet or a safe place, away from children or anyone with a history of substance abuse to prevent unauthorized access and potential misuse.

B) Correct: This statement reflects the nurse's understanding of the strategy to continuously assess for the development of tolerance and physical dependence when administering opioids over an extended period. Monitoring pain control and watching for signs of tolerance or dependence is crucial in opioid therapy.

C) Wrong: This statement is incorrect as it goes against the strategy of assessing the risk of GI bleeding associated with NSAID use, especially in patients with a history of ulcers or bleeding disorders. NSAIDs should be avoided in patients with a recent history of GI bleeding, as stated in the example.

D) Wrong: Administering naloxone as a preventive measure before opioid administration is not a standard practice. Naloxone is used to reverse opioid-induced respiratory depression in cases of overdose, not as a routine preventive measure.

E) Correct: This statement reflects the nurse's understanding of the strategy to consider individual pharmacogenetics when prescribing opioids. Altered drug metabolism due to genetic factors can impact the patient's response to opioids, and dose adjustments may be necessary.

F) Correct: This statement indicates that the nurse recognizes the importance of assessing for concurrent mental health issues in patients with chronic pain and a history of depression. A comprehensive pain management plan should include psychological support and monitoring for signs of worsening mental health.

G) Wrong: This statement is incorrect as it suggests escalating the opioid dose without monitoring for signs of tolerance or dependence. Opioid doses should be adjusted based on the patient's response and need, taking into account the risk of tolerance and dependence.

H) Wrong: Storing opioids in an accessible location within the home is not a safe practice, and this statement contradicts the strategy of educating patients on safe storage. Opioids should be kept in a secure, locked cabinet or safe place to prevent unauthorized access.

Antidepressants and anti-anxiety

NGN Case Study

Patient History:

Mr. Vimal, a 32-year-old male, presents to the emergency department (ED) with complaints of chest pain, shortness of breath, and dizziness. He reports a history of generalized anxiety disorder (GAD) and mentions that he has been under increased stress due to work-related issues.

Nurse Notes:

Upon assessment, Mr. Vimal appears restless, fidgety, and reports difficulty concentrating. He frequently checks his pulse and expresses fear of having a heart attack. He denies any recent trauma or substance use. The nurse observes increased muscle tension, rapid speech, and trembling hands.

Medication List and Doses:

Alprazolam (Xanax): 0.5 mg orally every 8 hours as needed for anxiety.

Escitalopram (Lexapro): 10 mg orally daily for generalized anxiety disorder.

Propranolol (Inderal): 20 mg orally every 12 hours as needed for palpitations.

Vital Signs:

Blood Pressure: 140/90 mmHg

Heart Rate: 110 bpm

Respiratory Rate: 20 breaths per minute

Temperature: 98.6°F (37°C)

Oxygen Saturation: 98% on room air

Lab Values:

Complete Blood Count (CBC):

WBC: 8,000/mm³

Hemoglobin: 13.5 g/dL

Platelets: 250,000/mm³

Basic Metabolic Panel (BMP):

Sodium: 138 mEq/L

Potassium: 4.2 mEq/L

Blood Urea Nitrogen (BUN): 18 mg/dL

Creatinine: 0.9 mg/dL

Glucose: 110 mg/dL

Que : Considering Mr. Vimal's symptoms and medical history, which medication is most likely contributing to his rapid speech and restlessness?

A) Alprazolam (Xanax)

B) Escitalopram (Lexapro)

C) Propranolol (Inderal)

D) None of the above

Escitalopram (Lexapro) is the one most likely to be associated with rapid speech and restlessness. Escitalopram is a selective serotonin reuptake inhibitor (SSRI) commonly used to treat depression and anxiety. While SSRIs are generally used to stabilize mood, they can sometimes cause activation symptoms, especially when starting treatment or adjusting dosages. These activation symptoms can include restlessness and increased energy, which might manifest as rapid speech.

Alprazolam (Xanax) is a benzodiazepine that typically has a calming effect and is used to treat anxiety. It is less likely to cause restlessness or rapid speech.

Propranolol (Inderal) is a beta-blocker used to manage symptoms of anxiety and is not typically associated with rapid speech or restlessness. It mainly affects physical symptoms of anxiety, like tremors and palpitations.

Que : Which of the following is a primary use for alprazolam?

A) Treating high blood pressure

B) Managing acute anxiety and panic disorders

C) Relieving chronic pain

D) Reducing inflammation

Answer: B) Managing acute anxiety and panic disorders

Explanation:

A) Treating high blood pressure

Explanation: Alprazolam is not used to treat high blood pressure. It is a benzodiazepine primarily used for its anxiolytic (anxiety-reducing) properties. High blood pressure is typically managed with medications like beta-blockers, ACE inhibitors, or diuretics, not benzodiazepines.

B) Managing acute anxiety and panic disorders

Explanation: This is the correct answer. Alprazolam is a benzodiazepine that is specifically prescribed to manage acute anxiety and panic disorders. It works by enhancing the effects of a neurotransmitter called gamma-aminobutyric acid (GABA) in the brain, which produces a calming effect. It is often used for short-term relief of severe anxiety symptoms and panic attacks.

C) Relieving chronic pain

Explanation: Alprazolam is not intended for pain management. Chronic pain is typically treated with analgesics, opioids, or non-opioid pain relievers, and sometimes adjunctive therapies like physical therapy or antidepressants. Alprazolam does not have pain-relieving properties and is not prescribed for pain management.

D) Reducing inflammation

Explanation: Alprazolam does not have anti-inflammatory properties. Inflammation is typically treated with nonsteroidal anti-inflammatory drugs (NSAIDs) or corticosteroids. Alprazolam is used for its anxiolytic effects and does not affect inflammation.

Que : In the nursing management of Mr. Vimal's anxiety, which of the following actions would be appropriate?

Options:

A) Administering a higher dose of Alprazolam (Xanax) to quickly alleviate his symptoms.

B) Encouraging Mr. Vimal to engage in deep-breathing exercises to help manage anxiety.

C) Advising Mr. Vimal to stop taking Escitalopram (Lexapro) immediately.

D) Suggesting that Mr. Vimal discontinue Propranolol (Inderal) to reduce restlessness.

E) Recommending an increase in the frequency of Alprazolam (Xanax) intake for better anxiety control.

F) Initiating a referral to a mental health professional for counseling and support.

G) Instructing Mr. Vimal to avoid any form of physical activity to minimize stress.

Ans :

Explanation:

The correct actions are B) Encouraging Mr. Vimal to engage in deep-breathing exercises to help manage anxiety and F) Initiating a referral to a mental health professional for counseling and support.

Explanation of Options:

A) Incorrect. Administering a higher dose of Alprazolam may not be appropriate and could lead to unwanted side effects.

B) Correct. Deep-breathing exercises are a non-pharmacological intervention to help manage anxiety.

C) Incorrect. Abruptly stopping Escitalopram (Lexapro) can lead to withdrawal symptoms, and any changes should be discussed with the healthcare provider.

D) Incorrect. Discontinuing Propranolol (Inderal) may not be advisable without consulting the healthcare provider, as it is prescribed for palpitations.

E) Incorrect. Increasing the frequency of Alprazolam (Xanax) intake without medical guidance can pose risks of dependence and side effects.

F) Correct. Referring Mr. Vimal to a mental health professional is appropriate for counseling and additional support.

G) Incorrect. Physical activity can be beneficial for managing stress, and avoiding it entirely is not recommended.

Que : Regarding the use of antianxiety medications, which statements are correct?

Options:

A) Alprazolam (Xanax) is a selective serotonin reuptake inhibitor (SSRI).

B) Escitalopram (Lexapro) is a benzodiazepine.

C) Propranolol (Inderal) primarily acts on the central nervous system to reduce anxiety.

D) Alprazolam (Xanax) should be abruptly stopped if side effects occur.

E) Escitalopram (Lexapro) may take several weeks to show its full therapeutic effect.

F) Propranolol (Inderal) is contraindicated in individuals with a history of palpitations.

G) Alprazolam (Xanax) may cause drowsiness and impair cognitive function.

H) Escitalopram (Lexapro) is commonly prescribed for immediate relief of acute anxiety.

Ans:

Explanation:

The correct statements are E) Escitalopram (Lexapro) may take several weeks to show its full therapeutic effect, G) Alprazolam (Xanax) may cause drowsiness and impair cognitive function

Explanation of Options:

A) Alprazolam (Xanax) is a selective serotonin reuptake inhibitor (SSRI).

Incorrect. Alprazolam is a benzodiazepine, not an SSRI. SSRIs, such as escitalopram (Lexapro), are used to treat anxiety and depression by increasing serotonin levels in the brain. Alprazolam, on the other hand, works by enhancing the effects of GABA, a neurotransmitter that produces a calming effect.

B) Escitalopram (Lexapro) is a benzodiazepine.

Incorrect. Escitalopram is an SSRI, not a benzodiazepine. SSRIs are used to treat anxiety and depression by increasing serotonin levels, whereas benzodiazepines, like alprazolam, are used for their sedative and anxiolytic effects.

C) Propranolol (Inderal) primarily acts on the central nervous system to reduce anxiety.

Incorrect. Propranolol is a beta-blocker that primarily affects the cardiovascular system by reducing heart rate and blood pressure. It is used to manage physical symptoms of anxiety, such as tremors and palpitations, but does not directly act on the central nervous system to reduce anxiety.

D) Alprazolam (Xanax) should be abruptly stopped if side effects occur.

Incorrect. Abruptly stopping alprazolam can lead to withdrawal symptoms, including increased anxiety, seizures, and other complications. It is generally recommended to taper off the medication gradually under medical supervision if discontinuation is necessary.

E) Escitalopram (Lexapro) may take several weeks to show its full therapeutic effect.

Correct. SSRIs like escitalopram typically take several weeks (often 4 to 6 weeks) to reach their full therapeutic effect. This delay is due to the time needed for serotonin levels to stabilize and produce noticeable improvements in mood and anxiety.

F) Propranolol (Inderal) is contraindicated in individuals with a history of palpitations.

Incorrect. Propranolol is actually used to manage palpitations and other symptoms of anxiety. It is not contraindicated for individuals with a history of palpitations; instead, it is often prescribed to help control these symptoms.

G) Alprazolam (Xanax) may cause drowsiness and impair cognitive function.

Correct. Alprazolam can cause drowsiness, dizziness, and cognitive impairment, particularly at higher doses or when first starting the medication. These side effects are common with benzodiazepines.

H) Escitalopram (Lexapro) is commonly prescribed for immediate relief of acute anxiety.

Incorrect. Escitalopram is not typically used for immediate relief of acute anxiety. SSRIs are more commonly prescribed for long-term management of anxiety and depression. For acute relief, benzodiazepines like alprazolam are usually preferred due to their faster onset of action.

Que : Which of the following physiological parameters is most likely to be affected by chronic stress?

A) Increased heart rate

B) Elevated platelet count

C) Decreased blood pressure

D) Reduced respiratory rate

Ans :

A) Increased heart rate

Right: Chronic stress activates the body's "fight or flight" response, leading to the release of stress hormones like adrenaline and cortisol. These hormones increase heart rate to prepare the body for immediate action.

B) Elevated platelet count

Wrong: While stress can affect various aspects of the immune system, it does not typically cause an elevated platelet count. Platelet count is more directly influenced by factors like bone marrow function, certain medications, and specific medical conditions.

C) Decreased blood pressure

Wrong: Chronic stress is more likely to cause increased blood pressure rather than decreased blood pressure. The stress response causes blood vessels to constrict and the heart to pump harder, which can raise blood pressure over time.

D) Reduced respiratory rate

Wrong: Chronic stress usually leads to an increased respiratory rate as part of the body's preparation for "fight or flight." Stress can cause rapid, shallow breathing, which is the opposite of a reduced respiratory rate.

Que : Read the following nurse's advice

Mr. Vimal, it's essential to address your anxiety symptoms effectively. Firstly, continue taking your prescribed medications as directed by your healthcare provider. Ensure that you are taking Alprazolam (Xanax) as needed for anxiety relief, Escitalopram (Lexapro) for your generalized anxiety disorder, and Propranolol (Inderal) as needed for palpitations. Secondly, consider incorporating relaxation techniques into your daily routine. Deep-breathing exercises and mindfulness can help alleviate stress. Additionally, maintaining a consistent sleep schedule is crucial for overall well-being, so aim for 7-9 hours of quality sleep each night. Moreover, try to identify and address specific stressors in your work environment, seeking support or making changes where possible. Regular physical activity is beneficial for both mental and physical health, so engage in activities you enjoy. Remember to stay hydrated and maintain a balanced diet to support your overall health. Lastly, if you notice any unusual side effects or worsening symptoms, promptly consult your healthcare provider for further guidance.

Que: Identify 2 Incorrect Sentences !

"Ensure that you are taking Alprazolam (Xanax) as needed for anxiety relief, Escitalopram (Lexapro) for your generalized anxiety disorder, and Propranolol (Inderal) as needed for palpitations."

Incorrect: Propranolol (Inderal) is not typically prescribed on an "as needed" basis for palpitations. It is usually taken regularly to manage symptoms.

"Alprazolam (Xanax) should be abruptly stopped if side effects occur."

Incorrect: Alprazolam (Xanax) should not be abruptly stopped due to the risk of withdrawal symptoms. It should be tapered off under medical supervision. The remaining recommendations about relaxation techniques, sleep, addressing stressors, physical activity, hydration, and diet are generally sound advice for managing anxiety and promoting overall well-being.

Anticoagulants and Antiplatelet

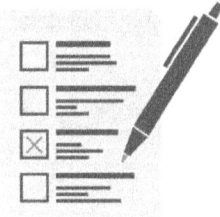 Anticoagulants, commonly known as blood thinners, inhibit blood clot formation, reducing the risk of stroke and heart attacks. Notable examples include aspirin, heparin, and warfarin, often encountered in exams. Nursing considerations include close monitoring of blood parameters, particularly platelet count, and recognition of potential side effects like bruising and gastrointestinal bleeding. Special caution is needed in patients with renal disorders as anticoagulants are primarily excreted through the kidneys. Warfarin, subject to a Black Box Warning, necessitates INR monitoring and avoidance of sudden dietary changes. Heparin, administered intravenously or subcutaneously, requires close monitoring for Heparin-Induced Thrombocytopenia (HIT). Aspirin, though effective, poses risks of peptic ulcers and bleeding, particularly in older individuals. Aspirin poisoning management involves activated charcoal and alkaline diuresis, with symptoms including dizziness and nausea. Its concurrent use with other anticoagulants or NSAIDs should be avoided due to increased bleeding risk.

Practice Session

Que: Anita is a 65-year-old woman who has been recently diagnosed with atrial fibrillation. Her healthcare provider has prescribed anticoagulant therapy to reduce her risk of stroke. Anita's nurse, Lisa, is responsible for educating her about the medication and its management.

During the education session, Lisa makes the following statements:

"You should take your anticoagulant medication with a full glass of grapefruit juice every morning."

"Anticoagulants work by preventing platelet aggregation in your blood vessels."

"It's essential to monitor your international normalized ratio (INR) regularly while taking anticoagulants."

Select which of the statements given by the nurse indicates that she doesn't know the correct information about anticoagulant therapy for atrial fibrillation?

A) Statement 1

B) Statement 2

C) Statement 3

D) Statement 1, 2 and 3

A) Statement 1: Incorrect Explanation: Statement 1 is incorrect. Patients should not take anticoagulant medications with grapefruit juice, as grapefruit juice can interfere with the metabolism of some drugs, potentially leading to higher drug levels in the blood. This statement indicates that the nurse lacks knowledge about the proper administration of anticoagulants.

B) Statement 2: Incorrect Explanation: Statement 2 is incorrect. Anticoagulants do not work by preventing platelet aggregation; they work by inhibiting clotting factors in the blood. This statement shows a misunderstanding of the mechanism of action of anticoagulants.

C) Statement 3: Correct Explanation: Statement 3 is correct. It is essential to monitor the international normalized ratio (INR) regularly while taking anticoagulants like warfarin. This monitoring helps ensure that the medication is working effectively and that the patient is within the desired therapeutic range to prevent clotting or bleeding complications. This statement demonstrates the nurse's knowledge of monitoring parameters for anticoagulant therapy.

D) All of the above: Incorrect Explanation: Statement D is incorrect because Statement 3 is correct. Therefore, not all the statements provided by the nurse indicate a lack of knowledge.

Que: Which of the following medications is primarily used to prevent blood clots in conditions like atrial fibrillation and deep vein thrombosis?

A) Heparin
B) Warfarin
C) Apixaban
D) Dabigatran
E) Rivaroxaban

Correct Answer: B) Warfarin (Coumadin)

Explanation of Each Option

A) Heparin

- **Why it's wrong:** Heparin is used for the prevention and treatment of blood clots, particularly in hospital settings, but it is typically administered for short-term management. It is often used for acute situations such as surgery or treatment of venous thromboembolism, but Warfarin is preferred for long-term anticoagulation, especially in outpatient management.

B) Warfarin

- **Why it's right:** Warfarin is specifically indicated for preventing blood clots in patients with atrial fibrillation, deep vein thrombosis, and pulmonary embolism. It works by inhibiting vitamin K-dependent clotting factors and is commonly used for long-term management.

C) Apixaban

- **Why it's wrong:** While Apixaban is also used to prevent blood clots in patients with atrial fibrillation and DVT, the question specifically asks for the medication that is primarily associated with this use, which is Warfarin. Apixaban is a newer anticoagulant and can be an alternative but is not the primary drug referenced in the context of traditional management.

D) Dabigatran

- **Why it's wrong:** Dabigatran is a direct thrombin inhibitor used to reduce the risk of stroke and systemic embolism in patients with non-valvular atrial fibrillation. Like Apixaban, it is effective but is not the primary medication traditionally used for the chronic management of these conditions as Warfarin is.

E) Rivaroxaban

- **Why it's wrong:** Rivaroxaban is another factor Xa inhibitor that is used to prevent blood clots in patients with atrial fibrillation and for treating DVT. However, it is not the first-line therapy when considering the historical context of anticoagulation treatment, which predominantly involves Warfarin.

Que: What is the primary clinical use of Warfarin (Coumadin)?

A) To treat acute coronary syndrome
B) To manage hypertension
C) To prevent blood clots in conditions like atrial fibrillation and deep vein thrombosis
D) To reduce symptoms of anxiety
E) To increase white blood cell count in patients with leukopenia

Correct Answer: C) To prevent blood clots in conditions like atrial fibrillation and deep vein thrombosis

Explanation of Each Option

A) To treat acute coronary syndrome

- **Why it's wrong:** While Warfarin may be used in some cases of coronary artery disease, it is not the first-line treatment for acute coronary syndrome (ACS). ACS typically requires antiplatelet medications like aspirin or clopidogrel for immediate management rather than anticoagulants like Warfarin.

B) To manage hypertension

- **Why it's wrong:** Warfarin is not used for managing hypertension. Antihypertensive medications, such as diuretics, ACE inhibitors, and beta-blockers, are used for that purpose. Warfarin is an anticoagulant, not an antihypertensive.

C) To prevent blood clots in conditions like atrial fibrillation and deep vein thrombosis

- **Why it's right:** Warfarin is primarily prescribed to prevent the formation of blood clots in patients with atrial fibrillation, deep vein thrombosis (DVT), and pulmonary embolism (PE). By inhibiting vitamin K-dependent clotting factors, it significantly reduces the risk of thromboembolic events.

D) To reduce symptoms of anxiety

- **Why it's wrong:** Warfarin is not indicated for the treatment of anxiety. Antianxiety medications, such as benzodiazepines and selective serotonin reuptake inhibitors (SSRIs), are used for this purpose. Warfarin's function is entirely related to anticoagulation.

E) To increase white blood cell count in patients with leukopenia

- **Why it's wrong:** Warfarin does not affect white blood cell counts. Medications that might be used to treat leukopenia include growth factors like granulocyte-colony stimulating factor (G-CSF). Warfarin is focused on anticoagulation, not hematopoiesis.

Cardiovascular medication

> **tip** Understand beta-blockers, calcium channel blockers, ACE inhibitors, ARBs, and diuretics, knowing their effects and side effects. For instance, metoprolol, a beta-blocker, can cause fatigue and bronchoconstriction.

Evaluate the patient's condition before medication administration. For instance, assess blood pressure before administering a calcium channel blocker like amlodipine.

Recognize potential interactions between cardiovascular medications and other drugs. Example: warfarin and amiodarone can increase bleeding risk.

Be vigilant for common adverse effects. Example: persistent dry cough with ACE inhibitors like lisinopril.

Administer medications accurately and educate patients. Example: educating about potential side effects of atorvastatin and lisinopril.

Assess patients for allergies or contraindications. Example: avoiding hydrochlorothiazide in patients allergic to sulfonamides.

Continuously assess the patient's response to medications. Example: assessing chest pain relief with nitroglycerin.

Consider how medications may affect pregnant or elderly patients. Example: discussing risks of labetalol in pregnant patients.

Assess and address diet, exercise, and smoking impacts. Example: discussing diet changes with patients prescribed atorvastatin.

Monitor for adverse effects associated with prolonged medication use. Example: monitoring for electrolyte imbalances with chronic diuretic use.

Assess patient understanding and compliance with medication regimens. Example: discussing the importance of regular blood tests with warfarin.

Understand when to use and avoid specific medications. Example: avoiding beta-blockers in patients with severe asthma.

Know different administration routes and implications. Example: administering nitroglycerin sublingually for rapid absorption.

Be familiar with dosage calculations for cardiovascular medications. Example: calculating digoxin dosage based on patient weight and condition.

Understand medication absorption, distribution, metabolism, and excretion. Example: recognizing the onset of action of furosemide.

Identify signs of medication toxicity and intervene appropriately. Example: recognizing signs of digoxin toxicity like nausea and vomiting.

Understand proper medication storage conditions. Example: storing nitroglycerin tablets away from heat and moisture.

Be aware of safe medication disposal methods. Example: advising patients to return expired medications to pharmacies.

Stay updated on new developments in cardiovascular medication management. Example: following recent guidelines for the use of direct oral anticoagulants.

Practice Session

Que: A 65-year-old male patient, Mr. Johnson, is admitted to the hospital with a diagnosis of heart failure. He has a history of hypertension and has been prescribed multiple cardiovascular medications. As the nurse responsible for his care, you must ensure safe medication administration and provide education to manage his condition effectively.

Select which of the statements given by the nurse indicates that they have effectively applied the principles of cardiovascular medication management for Mr. Johnson?

A. The nurse administers digoxin and emphasizes the importance of checking Mr. Johnson's blood pressure regularly.

B. The nurse assesses Mr. Johnson's heart rate before administering metoprolol and holds the medication when the heart rate is below 60 beats per minute.

C. The nurse reviews Mr. Johnson's medication list and notices he's taking warfarin and amiodarone; she administers both medications as scheduled.

D. The nurse educates Mr. Johnson about the potential side effect of dry cough associated with lisinopril and advises him to report it immediately.

E. The nurse administers amlodipine to Mr. Johnson without checking his blood pressure, as it's not necessary for this medication.

F. The nurse administers Mr. Johnson's diuretic medication in the evening to minimize disruptions to his daily routine.

G. The nurse administers Mr. Johnson's medications in one batch to save time during medication rounds.

H. The nurse advises Mr. Johnson to continue his medication regimen even if he experiences severe side effects, as stopping medications abruptly can be harmful.

Explanation:

A. **Incorrect**: While it's important to monitor Mr. Johnson's blood pressure regularly, digoxin is primarily used to treat heart failure by improving contractility and should not significantly affect blood pressure.

B. **Correct**: Assessing the patient's heart rate before administering metoprolol, a beta-blocker, is crucial. It is generally contraindicated to administer beta-blockers when the heart rate is below 60 beats per minute, as they can further slow the heart rate, potentially causing bradycardia or heart block.

C. **Incorrect**: Administering warfarin and amiodarone without considering potential drug interactions can increase the risk of bleeding. The nurse should consult with the healthcare provider or pharmacist to adjust the medication regimen if necessary.

D. **Correct**: Educating Mr. Johnson about the potential side effect of a dry cough associated with lisinopril (an ACE inhibitor) is important. This empowers the patient to recognize and report this side effect, potentially leading to a medication change if necessary.

E. **Incorrect**: Administering amlodipine without checking Mr. Johnson's blood pressure goes against the principle of assessing the patient's condition before medication administration. Blood pressure monitoring is essential when administering antihypertensive medications.

F. **Incorrect**: Administering diuretics in the evening may disrupt Mr. Johnson's sleep due to increased urination. The timing of diuretic administration should be carefully considered to minimize inconvenience to the patient.

G. **Incorrect**: Administering medications in one batch may save time but increases the risk of medication errors. Each medication should be administered separately and documented accurately.

H. **Correct**: Advising Mr. Johnson to continue his medication regimen even if he experiences severe side effects is crucial. Abruptly stopping cardiovascular medications can lead to rebound effects and worsen his condition. It's important to involve the healthcare provider in modifying the medication regimen if needed.

Antiarrhythmics

Memorize antiarrhythmics into four main classes: Class I (sodium channel blockers), Class II (beta blockers), Class III (potassium channel blockers), and Class IV (calcium channel blockers).

Class I antiarrhythmics include lidocaine and procainamide, which block sodium channels.

Class II antiarrhythmics, like propranolol and metoprolol, are beta blockers that reduce sympathetic stimulation.

Class III antiarrhythmics, including amiodarone and sotalol, prolong the repolarization phase by affecting potassium channels.

Class IV antiarrhythmics, such as verapamil and diltiazem, affect calcium channels, reducing heart rate and conduction.

Lidocaine can cause drowsiness, confusion, and seizures at high doses, with decreased effectiveness when combined with beta blockers.

Amiodarone may lead to pulmonary toxicity, thyroid dysfunction, and liver problems, with numerous potential drug interactions due to its long half-life.

Propranolol side effects include bradycardia, bronchoconstriction, and fatigue, with enhanced effects when combined with calcium channel blockers.

Verapamil side effects encompass bradycardia, constipation, and hypotension, with heightened effects in conjunction with beta blockers.

Grapefruit juice consumption can increase amiodarone levels due to CYP3A4 inhibition, leading to potential toxicity.

Herbal supplement use may pose interactions with antiarrhythmics, though not specific to amiodarone.

Cigarette smoking can affect medication metabolism but isn't a direct concern with amiodarone.

Exercise considerations like jogging should be assessed based on cardiac condition and healthcare provider recommendations.

Assess patient characteristics, including age and comorbidities, when prescribing antiarrhythmics like digoxin and flecainide.

Recognize emergency situations with antiarrhythmics, such as quinidine toxicity presenting with severe hypotension and widened QRS complexes.

Be proficient in dosage calculations for antiarrhythmics, ensuring accurate administration rates.

Interpret ECG changes associated with specific antiarrhythmics, such as prolonged QT intervals with sotalol.

Practice Session

A 65-year-old male patient, Mr. Johnson, is admitted to the cardiac care unit with a history of atrial fibrillation. He has been prescribed an antiarrhythmic medication, amiodarone, to control his arrhythmia. During the initial assessment, you notice certain habits and behaviors that could impact his medication management.

Patient Habits and Behaviors:

Mr. Johnson consumes grapefruit juice daily with breakfast.

He mentions taking herbal supplements he purchased online for overall health.

He admits to occasional cigarette smoking, typically a few cigarettes a day.

He expresses a desire to continue his daily jogging routine, even during his hospital stay.

Select which of the following habits of the patient suggests a potential concern or consideration in the administration of amiodarone?

A) Daily consumption of grapefruit juice.

B) Taking herbal supplements purchased online.

C) Occasional cigarette smoking.

D) Desire to continue jogging during the hospital stay.

Explanation: A) Daily consumption of grapefruit juice.

Correct Answer: A) Daily consumption of grapefruit juice.

Explanation: Daily consumption of grapefruit juice can be problematic when taking amiodarone. Grapefruit juice contains compounds that inhibit the enzyme CYP3A4, which plays a role in the metabolism of amiodarone. This inhibition can lead to increased levels of amiodarone in the bloodstream, potentially increasing the risk of side effects and toxicity.

B) Taking herbal supplements purchased online.

Explanation: While taking herbal supplements can raise concerns about potential interactions with prescribed medications, this option does not specifically relate to amiodarone. Therefore, it is not the primary concern in this case.

C) Occasional cigarette smoking.

Explanation: Cigarette smoking can affect the metabolism of certain medications by inducing hepatic enzymes. However, it is not a direct concern when taking amiodarone. Other factors in Mr. Johnson's case are more relevant.

D) Desire to continue jogging during the hospital stay.

Explanation: While exercise is an important aspect of overall health, the desire to continue jogging does not directly relate to amiodarone administration. However, it's essential to assess whether strenuous exercise is safe for Mr. Johnson based on his cardiac condition and the specific recommendations of his healthcare provider.

In this case, the correct answer is "A) Daily consumption of grapefruit juice" because it suggests a potential drug interaction concern when administering amiodarone. The nurse should educate

Cardiovascular drugs-digoxin

Practice Session

Que : Mrs. Ranjan is a 65-year-old woman who has been experiencing atrial fibrillation. Her doctor has prescribed her digoxin to help manage her heart rate and rhythm. However, Mrs. Ranjan has also been experiencing some side effects such as vomiting, diarrhea, and blurred vision.

What is the most likely cause of Mrs. Ranjan's side effects?

A) Hypokalemia

B) Hypercalcemia

C) Hypomagnesemia

D) Renal impairment

The most likely cause of Mrs. Ranjan's side effects, including vomiting, diarrhea, and blurred vision, is A) Hypokalemia.

Here's why each option is considered:

A) Hypokalemia

Correct. Digoxin has a narrow therapeutic window and its effectiveness and toxicity are closely related to potassium levels in the body. Hypokalemia (low potassium levels) can increase the risk of digoxin toxicity, leading to symptoms such as vomiting, diarrhea, and blurred vision. These symptoms are classic signs of digoxin toxicity.

B) Hypercalcemia

Less likely. While hypercalcemia can affect digoxin toxicity, it is not as commonly associated with the specific symptoms of vomiting, diarrhea, and blurred vision. Hypercalcemia typically affects the heart rhythm but is less directly related to the symptoms described.

C) Hypomagnesemia

Less likely. Hypomagnesemia (low magnesium levels) can also increase the risk of digoxin toxicity, but it is more commonly associated with arrhythmias and not directly with gastrointestinal symptoms like vomiting and diarrhea.

D) Renal impairment

Less likely. Renal impairment can affect digoxin levels and lead to toxicity since digoxin is primarily excreted by the kidneys. However, the specific symptoms described are more directly related to electrolyte imbalances like hypokalemia rather than renal impairment alone. Nonetheless, renal impairment can also contribute to digoxin toxicity if it leads to elevated drug levels.

Explanation: It is important to remember that digoxin can cause electrolyte imbalance, particularly hypokalemia, which can lead to various symptoms such as vomiting, diarrhea, and blurred vision. It is also important to monitor digoxin levels in patients with renal impairment, electrolyte imbalance, and elderly patients, as they may be more prone to experiencing side effects. In addition, digoxin can compete with other drugs for renal clearance, which may lead to increased side effects of those drugs. It is used to treat heart conditions with high impulse rates, such as atrial flutter and atrial fibrillation, by slowing down the heart rate, but if not monitored carefully, it can also cause bradycardia.

Antidiabetic medication

Insulin is the preferred treatment for gestational diabetes during pregnancy due to its safety profile and inability to cross the placenta.

Oral hypoglycemic agents include sulfonylureas, biguanides, thiazolidinediones, alpha-glucosidase inhibitors, DPP-4 inhibitors, and SGLT2 inhibitors.

Sulfonylureas stimulate the pancreas to release insulin and may interact with antibiotics and NSAIDs.

Biguanides like metformin reduce glucose production by the liver and improve insulin sensitivity but may cause gastrointestinal upset and rare lactic acidosis.

Thiazolidinediones improve insulin sensitivity but can lead to fluid retention and weight gain.

Alpha-glucosidase inhibitors slow carbohydrate absorption in the intestines and may cause gastrointestinal upset.

DPP-4 inhibitors enhance incretin hormones to stimulate insulin release with few interactions.

SGLT2 inhibitors promote glucose excretion in urine but may increase the risk of urinary tract infections and hypotension.

Patient education should emphasize medication adherence to prevent uncontrolled blood glucose levels.

Proper insulin administration techniques, including injection sites and rotation, are essential for effective treatment.

Regular blood glucose monitoring is crucial to assess glycemic control and adjust treatment as needed.

Patients should be educated about signs of hypoglycemia and hyperglycemia and how to respond appropriately.

Gestational diabetes requires careful management during pregnancy, often with adjustments to medication regimens.

Insulin is the safest option for managing blood sugar levels during pregnancy and is preferred over oral medications.

Medication storage and handling should follow manufacturer instructions to maintain efficacy and safety, especially for insulin.

Practice Session

Que : Mary is a 45-year-old woman who has recently been diagnosed with type 2 diabetes mellitus. Her healthcare provider has prescribed antidiabetic medication as part of her treatment plan. Mary is eager to learn about her medications and how to manage her condition effectively. She seeks guidance from her nurse to ensure her safety and well-being.

Select which of the following scenarios suggests appropriate patient education regarding antidiabetic medications:

A. Mary is instructed to take her metformin on an empty stomach to maximize its absorption.

B. Mary is advised to monitor her blood glucose levels only when she experiences symptoms of hypoglycemia.

C. Mary is educated on the importance of adhering to her medication regimen and the potential consequences of missed doses.

D. Mary is encouraged to consume a high-sugar diet to prevent hypoglycemia while taking insulin.

E. Mary is informed that she can discontinue her antidiabetic medications once her blood glucose levels stabilize.

F. Mary is told that physical activity has no impact on blood glucose control and can be ignored.

G. Mary is advised to store her insulin vials in the freezer to prolong their shelf life.

H. Mary is instructed to administer her GLP-1 receptor agonist injection immediately before her meals.

Explanation:

C. Mary is educated on the importance of adhering to her medication regimen and the potential consequences of missed doses.

This scenario suggests appropriate patient education because it emphasizes medication adherence, a crucial aspect of diabetes management. Skipping doses can lead to uncontrolled blood glucose levels, so educating Mary about this is essential.

H. Mary is instructed to administer her GLP-1 receptor agonist injection immediately before her meals.

This scenario is also correct as it aligns with the proper administration technique for GLP-1 receptor agonists, which should be administered before meals to enhance their effectiveness in controlling postprandial blood glucose levels.

Now, let's explain why the other options are incorrect:

A. Mary is instructed to take her metformin on an empty stomach to maximize its absorption.

This is incorrect because metformin should be taken with meals to reduce the risk of gastrointestinal side effects.

B. Mary is advised to monitor her blood glucose levels only when she experiences symptoms of hypoglycemia.

This is incorrect because blood glucose monitoring should be regular and not limited to only when symptoms of hypoglycemia occur. Monitoring is essential to assess glycemic control and adjust treatment as needed.

D. Mary is encouraged to consume a high-sugar diet to prevent hypoglycemia while taking insulin.

This is incorrect as consuming a high-sugar diet can lead to hyperglycemia, not prevent hypoglycemia. Patients on insulin should manage their carbohydrate intake and balance it with their insulin doses.

E. Mary is informed that she can discontinue her antidiabetic medications once her blood glucose levels stabilize.

This is incorrect because type 2 diabetes typically requires ongoing management, and discontinuing medications without medical guidance can lead to worsened glycemic control.

F. Mary is told that physical activity has no impact on blood glucose control and can be ignored.

This is incorrect because physical activity is an essential component of diabetes management as it helps improve insulin sensitivity and blood glucose control.

G. Mary is advised to store her insulin vials in the freezer to prolong their shelf life.

This is incorrect because insulin should not be stored in the freezer. It should be stored in a refrigerator or at room temperature, as per the manufacturer's instructions, to maintain its effectiveness.

Que: A 45-year-old male patient, Mr. Johnson, has been recently diagnosed with type 2 diabetes mellitus. He presents to the clinic with complaints of increased thirst, frequent urination, and unexplained weight loss over the past few months. After confirming the diagnosis, the nurse initiates a discussion with Mr. Johnson regarding his condition and the necessary steps for self-management. During the conversation, Mr. Johnson becomes visibly anxious and expresses concerns about his ability to manage diabetes effectively. He mentions feeling overwhelmed and fearful of complications.

Select which of the following statements from a nurse needs to provide appropriate psychosocial support and address Mr. Johnson's mental health concerns:

A) "Mr. Johnson, diabetes is a common condition, and many people manage it successfully. You'll be fine." B) "I can see that you're feeling anxious, Mr. Johnson. Let's talk more about your concerns and explore ways to manage your anxiety." C) "Don't worry, Mr. Johnson. We have excellent medications to control your blood sugar levels. You don't need to stress." D) "Mr. Johnson, I understand you're concerned, but let's focus on the diet plan for now, and we can address your anxiety later."

Explanation:

B) "I can see that you're feeling anxious, Mr. Johnson. Let's talk more about your concerns and explore ways to manage your anxiety." - This statement is the correct choice because it acknowledges Mr. Johnson's anxiety and opens the door for further discussion and support. Addressing the patient's emotional needs is essential in providing psychosocial support.

A) "Mr. Johnson, diabetes is a common condition, and many people manage it successfully. You'll be fine." - While this statement is reassuring, it does not directly address Mr. Johnson's current emotional state or provide a pathway for managing his anxiety.

C) "Don't worry, Mr. Johnson. We have excellent medications to control your blood sugar levels. You don't need to stress." - This statement focuses solely on medication and dismisses Mr. Johnson's anxiety. It does not offer emotional support.

D) "Mr. Johnson, I understand you're concerned, but let's focus on the diet plan for now, and we can address your anxiety later." - This statement delays addressing Mr. Johnson's anxiety, which may worsen his distress. It's important to address psychological concerns promptly.

Que: Mr. B is a 50-year-old man who was recently diagnosed with type 1 diabetes. He is struggling to cope with his new diagnosis and is feeling overwhelmed by the daily management of insulin injections. He has a history of anxiety and depression. As his nurse, what is the most important nursing intervention for Mr. B in this situation?

a) Teaching him to skip insulin injections when he feels too stressed

b) Providing emotional support and addressing his anxiety and depression

c) Recommending he switch to an oral medication for diabetes

d) Encouraging him to eat sugary snacks to alleviate his anxiety

Answer:

b) Providing emotional support and addressing his anxiety and depression

Rationale:

The correct answer is b) Providing emotional support and addressing his anxiety and depression. It is crucial to prioritize Mr. B's mental and emotional well-being, especially given his history of anxiety and depression. Managing diabetes, particularly with insulin injections, can be overwhelming, and addressing his emotional health will be essential in helping him cope with his new diagnosis and daily management.

Explanation:

Option a) Teaching him to skip insulin injections when he feels too stressed is incorrect because skipping insulin injections can lead to uncontrolled blood sugar levels and complications. It's essential to find strategies to help him manage stress without compromising his diabetes management.

Option c) Recommending he switch to an oral medication for diabetes is incorrect because type 1 diabetes typically requires insulin therapy, and oral medications are not a suitable alternative for managing this type of diabetes.

Option d) Encouraging him to eat sugary snacks to alleviate his anxiety is incorrect because consuming sugary snacks can lead to blood sugar spikes and is not a recommended strategy for managing diabetes. It is important to address the root causes of his anxiety and provide healthier coping mechanisms.

Que: A patient with type 2 diabetes is prescribed insulin as part of their treatment plan. The patient is also a heavy drinker, frequently consuming alcohol on a daily basis. The patient is scheduled to undergo a contrast test for cardiac catheterization in the near future.

What is the best course of action for the patient in regards to their insulin prescription?

A) Continue taking insulin as prescribed, even if the patient consumes alcohol.

B) Tell the patient to stop consuming alcohol while taking insulin.

C) Stop taking insulin 48 hours before the contrast test.

D) Supplement the patient with vitamin D while taking insulin.

Answer:

B) Tell the patient to stop consuming alcohol while taking insulin.

Rationale:

Alcohol consumption while taking insulin can lead to unpredictable fluctuations in blood sugar levels. It can both increase the risk of hypoglycemia (low blood sugar) and, in some cases, mask the symptoms of hypoglycemia. Therefore, the best course of action would be to tell the patient to stop consuming alcohol while taking insulin. Option A is incorrect because consuming alcohol with insulin is not advisable. Option C is incorrect because it is not related to the patient's alcohol consumption. Option D is incorrect because supplementing with vitamin D is not the most pressing concern in this case, and it is not directly related to insulin use.

Explanation: Just like in the case of metformin, alcohol should not be consumed while taking insulin due to the potential risk of dangerous fluctuations in blood sugar levels. This is the primary concern, and addressing the patient's alcohol consumption is the most appropriate course of action.

Que : A patient with type 2 diabetes is prescribed metformin as the first-line treatment. The patient is a 65-year-old smoker with a history of renal disease. During the first week of treatment, the patient experiences diarrhea, gastrointestinal disturbance, and a metallic taste in their mouth. The patient also reports feeling weak, with bradycardia, hypotension, and lethargy.

Which of the following is a potential side effect of metformin treatment in a patient with type 2 diabetes?

A) Hypoglycemia

B) Lactic acidosis

C) Vitamin B12 deficiency

D) Liver failure

Rationale: Metformin is associated with several side effects, and the symptoms described can be linked to these potential issues. Here's a breakdown of each option:

A) Hypoglycemia

Less common. Metformin itself typically does not cause hypoglycemia, though it can enhance the effects of other glucose-lowering medications that might lead to hypoglycemia.

B) Lactic acidosis

Correct. Lactic acidosis is a rare but serious side effect of metformin, particularly in patients with renal impairment or other risk factors. Symptoms like weakness, bradycardia, hypotension, and lethargy could be indicative of lactic acidosis, which requires prompt medical attention.

C) Vitamin B12 deficiency

Correct. Metformin use is associated with vitamin B12 deficiency, which can develop over time and may contribute to fatigue and weakness. Regular monitoring of vitamin B12 levels is recommended for long-term metformin users.

D) Liver failure

Incorrect. Liver failure is not a common or known side effect of metformin. While liver function should be monitored, particularly in patients with pre-existing liver conditions, liver failure itself is not a typical side effect of metformin.

Psychotropic Medications

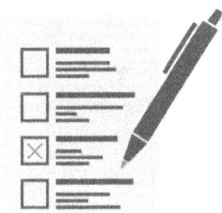
In psychiatric nursing, ensuring safe and effective medication management is paramount for patients with mental health disorders. This involves a multifaceted approach that includes thorough assessment, patient education, therapeutic communication, and cultural competence. Nurses must consider the patient's medical history, allergies, and potential drug interactions before administering psychotropic medications. Patient education plays a crucial role in promoting medication adherence and empowering patients to actively participate in their treatment plans. Regular follow-up appointments allow for ongoing assessment of medication effectiveness, side effects, and the need for adjustments. Additionally, monitoring for signs of withdrawal, drug tolerance, or resistance is essential to prevent adverse outcomes and ensure continued treatment efficacy. Collaboration with patients, their families, and interdisciplinary teams facilitates holistic care and addresses individual needs and preferences. By adhering to evidence-based practices and fostering open communication, psychiatric nurses can optimize patient outcomes and promote mental health and well-being.

Practice Session

Case Study:

A 35-year-old male patient with a history of schizophrenia is admitted to a psychiatric unit due to worsening agitation and aggressive behavior. The healthcare team decides to administer a psychotropic medication to help manage his symptoms. As the nurse assigned to this patient, you need to follow best practices when considering medication interventions.

Que : Select which of the following statements from a nurse needs to be followed when administering psychotropic medication to the patient:

A) Administer the medication immediately to address the agitation.

B) Understand the patient's medical history and allergies.

C) Provide the medication without discussing potential side effects.

D) Administer the medication without obtaining informed consent.

Explanation:

A) Administer the medication immediately to address the agitation.

Wrong: This option is incorrect. The nurse should not rush to administer medication without first assessing the patient's condition and needs, as mentioned in the case study. Assessing the patient's mental status, vital signs, and potential triggers for agitation is essential before any intervention.

B) Understand the patient's medical history and allergies.

Right: This option is correct. It aligns with the strategy of understanding the patient's condition and needs before medication administration. Knowing the patient's medical history and allergies is crucial to ensure safe medication administration and avoid potential contraindications or adverse reactions.

C) Provide the medication without discussing potential side effects.

Wrong: This option is incorrect. Patient education and informed consent are essential aspects of administering psychotropic medications. Patients have the right to know about potential side effects, benefits, and alternatives before treatment.

D) Administer the medication without obtaining informed consent.

Wrong: This option is incorrect. Even in situations where patients may lack decision-making capacity, obtaining informed consent from a legal guardian or authorized representative is crucial, as mentioned in the case study. It respects the patient's rights and ensures ethical and legal practice.

Que: Which class of medications is primarily used to treat depression by increasing neurotransmitter levels in the brain?

A) Antianxiety Medications

B) Antipsychotics

C) Mood Stabilizers

D) Stimulants

E) Antidepressants

Correct Answer: E) Antidepressants

A) Antianxiety Medications

Why it's wrong: Antianxiety medications, such as benzodiazepines, are primarily used to reduce anxiety symptoms. They work by enhancing the effect of the neurotransmitter GABA, which helps to calm the nervous system. While they may be prescribed for some individuals who also experience depression, they do not directly increase neurotransmitter levels associated with depression, like serotonin and norepinephrine.

B) Antipsychotics

Why it's wrong: Antipsychotics are used to manage symptoms of schizophrenia and bipolar disorder. They primarily alter the effects of dopamine and other neurotransmitters in the brain, which can help with mood stabilization but are not primarily designed to treat depression. Some atypical antipsychotics may have antidepressant effects and can be used as adjuncts in treatment-resistant depression, but they are not the first-line treatment for depression itself.

C) Mood Stabilizers

Why it's wrong: Mood stabilizers, such as lithium and anticonvulsants, are mainly used to manage mood swings, particularly in bipolar disorder. They help stabilize mood and prevent the extremes of mania and depression but do not primarily increase serotonin or norepinephrine levels to treat depressive episodes.

D) Stimulants

Why it's wrong: Stimulants are often prescribed for Attention Deficit Hyperactivity Disorder (ADHD) and work by increasing the levels of neurotransmitters like dopamine and norepinephrine. While some studies suggest that certain stimulants may have mood-enhancing effects, they are not primarily used to treat depression. Their main focus is on improving attention and focus rather than treating depressive symptoms.

E) Antidepressants

Why it's right: Antidepressants, specifically selective serotonin reuptake inhibitors (SSRIs) and serotonin-norepinephrine reuptake inhibitors (SNRIs), are the primary class of medications used to treat depression. They work by increasing the levels of neurotransmitters such as serotonin and norepinephrine in the brain, which are often found to be imbalanced in individuals with depression. This class of medication is designed specifically to alleviate the symptoms of depression and improve overall mood.

Antiemetics and Gastrointestinal drugs

Proton Pump Inhibitors (PPIs):

Examples: Omeprazole, Lansoprazole

Purpose: Reduce stomach acid production.

Side Effects: Long-term use can lead to low magnesium levels and increase the risk of fractures.

Remember: "PPIs put the P in Pump, reducing acid P-roduction."

H2-Receptor Antagonists:

Examples: Ranitidine, Famotidine

Purpose: Reduce stomach acid production (not as strong as PPIs).

Side Effects: Rarely, can cause confusion and arrhythmias.

Remember: "H2 blockers keep the H2 in check, but they're not as strong as PPIs."

Antiemetics (for nausea and vomiting):

Examples: Ondansetron (Zofran), Metoclopramide (Reglan)

Purpose: Prevent or relieve nausea and vomiting.

Side Effects: Ondansetron: Headache, constipation. Metoclopramide: Restlessness, drowsiness.

Remember: "Antiemetics end the 'A-Nausea' party."

Antacids:

Examples: Tums, Maalox

Purpose: Provide quick relief for heartburn and indigestion.

Side Effects: Can cause constipation (calcium-based) or diarrhea (magnesium-based).

Remember: "Antacids are like Tums for your tummy."

Laxatives:

Examples: Bisacodyl, Psyllium

Purpose: Promote bowel movements.

Side Effects: Overuse can lead to dependency and electrolyte imbalances.

Remember: "Laxatives help you 'let go,' but don't let them take control."

Anti-Diarrheal:

Examples: Loperamide (Imodium)

Purpose: Slows down diarrhea.

Side Effects: Constipation if overused.

Remember: "Loperamide locks the 'loose' door."

Gastric Protectants (for ulcers):

Examples: Sucralfate

Purpose: Forms a protective coating over ulcers.

Side Effects: Minimal, but can interfere with other medication absorption.

Remember: "Sucralfate shields your stomach like a 'sugar-surfboard.'"

Drug Interactions Tip: Be cautious with antacids and other medications. Antacids can affect the absorption of other drugs. Take them at least 1-2 hours apart from other medications.

Practice Session

Mrs. Anderson, a 55-year-old woman, presents to the emergency department with complaints of severe nausea and vomiting. She reports a history of gastritis and is currently taking several medications for various health conditions. The healthcare team suspects that her symptoms are related to her medication regimen and gastrointestinal issues.

Que : Select which of the following practices is NOT related to the safe and effective management of medications for gastrointestinal distress in Mrs. Anderson's case?

A) Understanding the major classes of antiemetics and gastrointestinal medications.

B) Knowing when to administer medications based on Mrs. Anderson's symptoms.

C) Being aware of common side effects and adverse reactions associated with these medications.

D) Safely calculating and administering the correct dosage of prescribed medications.

E) Providing patient education on the timing and interaction of medications with food and other drugs.

Explanation:

A) Understanding the major classes of antiemetics and gastrointestinal medications is crucial in this case because it helps healthcare providers identify potential causes of Mrs. Anderson's symptoms and choose appropriate treatments. This practice is relevant to her care and should be employed.

B) Knowing when to administer medications based on Mrs. Anderson's symptoms is essential. Administering medications at the right time can alleviate her symptoms effectively. This practice is relevant and important for her care.

C) Being aware of common side effects and adverse reactions associated with these medications is critical to monitor Mrs. Anderson's condition. Identifying adverse reactions promptly ensures her safety and well-being. This practice is relevant and important for her care.

D) Safely calculating and administering the correct dosage of prescribed medications is fundamental to prevent medication errors and ensure that Mrs. Anderson receives the appropriate treatment. This practice is highly relevant and crucial for her care.

E) Providing patient education on the timing and interaction of medications with food and other drugs is important to ensure Mrs. Anderson's understanding of her medication regimen. It helps her take her medications correctly and avoid potential interactions. This practice is relevant and important for her care.

Answer: B) Knowing when to administer medications based on Mrs. Anderson's symptoms.

In this case, Mrs. Anderson's symptoms are severe nausea and vomiting, which indicate an immediate need for intervention. Knowing when to administer medications in response to her symptoms is a critical aspect of her care, making option B the correct answer.

Option B is not relevant because it is vital to understand when and how to administer medications for symptom relief in gastrointestinal distress cases like Mrs. Anderson's.

Anita has completed her course of antiemetic medication. What instructions should the nurse provide regarding medication disposal?

A) Advise Anita to flush the unused medication down the toilet.

B) Instruct Anita to keep it for future use.

C) Tell Anita to throw it in the regular trash.

D) Recommend that Anita return it to a pharmacy or drug take-back program.

Explanation: A) Incorrect. Flushing unused medication down the toilet is not a safe method of disposal as it can lead to environmental contamination. B) Incorrect. Keeping unused medication for future use is not recommended as it may pose safety risks or lead to the inappropriate use of medication. C) Incorrect. Throwing medication in the regular trash can potentially lead to accidental ingestion by others or environmental contamination. D) Correct. Recommending that Anita return unused medications to a pharmacy or drug take-back program is the safest and most responsible way to dispose of medication. It helps prevent accidental ingestion, misuse, and environmental harm.

Antihypertensives

> **tip** Understanding antihypertensive medications is crucial for effective patient care. Diuretics, such as Hydrochlorothiazide and Furosemide, promote frequent urination and may lead to hypokalemia. Beta-blockers like Metoprolol and Atenolol can cause bradycardia and fatigue, with potential interactions affecting asthmatic and diabetic patients. ACE inhibitors such as Lisinopril and Enalapril are known for persistent cough and hyperkalemia, while ARBs like Losartan and Valsartan offer a safer alternative, especially during pregnancy. Calcium channel blockers such as Amlodipine and Verapamil can induce peripheral edema and constipation. Alpha-blockers like Doxazosin and Prazosin may result in orthostatic hypotension, while central alpha agonists like Clonidine and Methyldopa cause sedation and dry mouth, necessitating caution in discontinuation. Direct vasodilators like Hydralazine can lead to reflex tachycardia and headaches. Remembering key characteristics aids in medication management, including diuretics for fluid elimination, beta-blockers for heart rate control, ACE inhibitors/ARBs for cough avoidance and potassium elevation, calcium channel blockers for constipation and edema, alpha-blockers for orthostatic hypotension, central alpha agonists for gradual cessation, and direct vasodilators for headache and heart rate elevation. Understanding mechanisms, recognizing side effects, considering indications and contraindications, monitoring for interactions, assessing patient response, and differentiating between first-line and second-line agents are essential strategies for effective management and patient safety.

Practice Session

Que : Anita, a 55-year-old woman, visits her primary care physician complaining of persistent high blood pressure readings. After a thorough evaluation, her physician prescribes an antihypertensive medication. As her nurse, you need to ensure that Anita understands her medication and its potential side effects.

Scenario: Anita has been prescribed an antihypertensive medication due to her elevated blood pressure. She is given a prescription for lisinopril, an ACE inhibitor. Anita expresses concerns about potential side effects and how the medication works.

What should be your response to Anita's concerns about lisinopril, an ACE inhibitor?

A) Explain that ACE inhibitors work by blocking calcium channels in cardiac and smooth muscle cells.

B) Reassure Anita that lisinopril is a beta-blocker and has a low risk of side effects.

C) Advise Anita to monitor her blood pressure only once a week since ACE inhibitors rarely cause side effects.

D) Recommend discontinuing the medication immediately if she experiences a dry cough.

Explanation:

A) Incorrect. ACE inhibitors do not primarily work by blocking calcium channels. The correct mechanism of action is inhibiting the conversion of angiotensin I to angiotensin II.

B) Incorrect. Lisinopril is not a beta-blocker; it is an ACE inhibitor. Providing incorrect information can lead to confusion.

C) Incorrect. ACE inhibitors, including lisinopril, can have side effects, and patients should monitor their blood pressure regularly. This option provides inaccurate information.

D) Correct. ACE inhibitors like lisinopril are known to cause a persistent dry cough in some patients. If Anita experiences this side effect, it is appropriate to recommend discontinuing the medication and consulting with her healthcare provider. This action ensures patient safety and adherence to medication.

In this case, option D is the correct response because it addresses the potential side effect associated with ACE inhibitors and advises the patient on the appropriate course of action.

Que : Mary, a 58-year-old woman, has been diagnosed with hypertension during a routine checkup at her primary care physician's office. Her blood pressure readings consistently range around 160/100 mm Hg. After discussing her medical history and assessing her overall health, Mary's physician prescribes an antihypertensive medication to help manage her blood pressure. Mary has a history of sulfa drug allergy and is concerned about potential allergic reactions. She is also curious about what lifestyle changes she should consider. Mary's nurse provides her with education and reassurance regarding her treatment plan.

Which of the following habits of the patient is essential to consider when managing her hypertension and antihypertensive medication?

A) Assessing her dietary preferences and encouraging high-sodium foods.

B) Recognizing hypertensive emergencies and self-administering antihypertensive medications.

C) Ignoring potential allergies, as antihypertensive medications do not typically cause allergic reactions.

D) Considering lifestyle modifications, including dietary changes, exercise, and stress management.

E) Monitoring her cholesterol levels to manage hypertension effectively.

F) Monitoring her hemoglobin levels for signs of anemia.

G) Monitoring her calcium levels due to potential interactions with antihypertensive medications.

H) Monitoring her blood glucose levels to prevent hypoglycemia.

Explanation:

A) Incorrect: Assessing dietary preferences is essential, but encouraging high-sodium foods is counterproductive for managing hypertension. The correct approach is to recommend a low-sodium diet.

B) Incorrect: While recognizing hypertensive emergencies is crucial, self-administering antihypertensive medications without healthcare guidance is not advisable. It's a healthcare provider's responsibility to administer these medications.

C) Incorrect: This statement is false. Antihypertensive medications can indeed cause allergic reactions, especially in individuals with known allergies.

D) Correct: Lifestyle modifications, including dietary changes, exercise, and stress management, play a significant role in managing hypertension effectively. This aligns with the nursing strategy mentioned.

E) Incorrect: Monitoring cholesterol levels is essential for overall cardiovascular health but not directly related to the management of hypertension.

F) Incorrect: Monitoring hemoglobin levels is unrelated to the management of hypertension.

G) Incorrect: Monitoring calcium levels is generally not a primary concern when managing hypertension with antihypertensive medications. It's more crucial to monitor electrolyte levels like potassium.

H) Incorrect: Monitoring blood glucose levels is important for individuals with diabetes but not a primary concern in managing hypertension.

Que: Mr. Patel, a 55-year-old man, has been diagnosed with hypertension, and his doctor has prescribed him an antihypertensive medication, enalapril, an ACE inhibitor. After taking the medication for a few weeks, Mr. Patel experiences a persistent dry cough. He is concerned about this side effect and is unsure whether he should continue taking the medication.

What is a potential side effect of taking an ACE inhibitor like enalapril?

a) Swelling of the ankles and legs

b) Weight gain

c) Persistent dry cough

d) Hypoglycemia

Answer: c) Persistent dry cough

Rationale: The correct answer is c) persistent dry cough. ACE inhibitors, including enalapril, can cause a bothersome side effect of a persistent dry cough in some individuals. This is an important side effect to be aware of, and patients should discuss it with their healthcare provider. Options a) swelling of the ankles and legs and b) weight gain are more commonly associated with other types of antihypertensive medications. Option d) hypoglycemia is not a typical side effect of ACE inhibitors.

Explanation: ACE inhibitors work by relaxing blood vessels and helping to lower blood pressure. However, they can also lead to the development of a dry cough in some individuals, which may require a change in medication or further evaluation by a healthcare provider. Patients prescribed ACE inhibitors should communicate any unusual symptoms or side effects to their healthcare professional for proper management.

Que: Which class of antihypertensive drugs is often used as a first-line treatment for hypertension?

A) Beta Blockers

B) Calcium Channel Blockers

C) Diuretics

D) Renin Inhibitors

Correct Answer: C) Diuretics

Explanation:

A) Beta Blockers: Typically not the first-line treatment for hypertension; they're often used in patients with other cardiovascular conditions.

B) Calcium Channel Blockers: Effective but not usually the first choice in treating hypertension.

C) Diuretics: Correct answer. They are often the first-line treatment for hypertension due to their effectiveness in reducing blood volume.

D) Renin Inhibitors: Not commonly used as first-line therapy for hypertension.

Que: True/False

ACE inhibitors can cause a persistent dry cough.

Answer: True

Explanation: ACE inhibitors, such as Lisinopril and Enalapril, can lead to a persistent dry cough in some patients due to the accumulation of bradykinin. This is a common side effect of this class of medications.

Que: Fill in the Blank

Calcium Channel Blockers work by inhibiting calcium ions from entering _____ and _____ muscle cells, leading to vasodilation.

Answer: cardiac; smooth

Explanation: Calcium Channel Blockers, like Amlodipine and Diltiazem, inhibit calcium ions from entering cardiac and smooth muscle cells. This action causes relaxation and dilation of blood vessels, which helps to reduce blood pressure.

Diuretics

> ✓ All diuretics help in throwing out sodium and water so basically in toxic doses all diuretics cases dehydration.
> ✓ All diuretics can induce digoxin toxicity except for potassium-sparing diuretics
> ✓ All diuretics are contraindicated in patients with lithium and this can cause lithium toxicity.

Understanding diuretics is essential for safe and effective patient care. Diuretics increase urine production through various mechanisms, such as blocking sodium and chloride reabsorption in the kidneys' loops of Henle. They are indicated for conditions like hypertension and heart failure but must be used cautiously in patients with renal failure due to potential adverse effects. Diuretics can lead to electrolyte imbalances and dehydration, necessitating vigilant monitoring for signs like hypokalemia and hyponatremia. Additionally, diuretics can interact with medications like NSAIDs, increasing the risk of renal dysfunction. It's crucial to recognize potassium-sparing diuretics, which do not induce digoxin toxicity, and be aware of contraindications such as lithium use, which can lead to lithium toxicity. Nurses play a vital role in diuretic therapy by assessing for dehydration signs, monitoring vital signs, and evaluating electrolyte levels. Familiarity with both brand and generic names enhances medication identification and administration accuracy, contributing to patient safety. Applying knowledge to clinical scenarios ensures effective patient care and promotes optimal outcomes in diuretic therapy.

Patient Profile:

- Name: Mrs. Johnson
- Age: 62
- Medical History: Hypertension, type 2 diabetes, chronic kidney disease (CKD) stage 2
- Current Medications: Lisinopril, hydrochlorothiazide (HCTZ), metformin

Clinical Scenario: Mrs. Johnson presents for her routine follow-up appointment. During the visit, the nurse reviews her medication adherence, dietary habits, and any side effects she may have experienced since starting hydrochlorothiazide for her hypertension.

Which statement made by the nurse is correct regarding Mrs. Johnson's treatment with hydrochlorothiazide?

A) Hydrochlorothiazide can cause you to lose potassium; be sure to eat potassium-rich foods like bananas.
B) It's essential to monitor your blood pressure daily, especially since you're taking hydrochlorothiazide.
C) Since you have chronic kidney disease, I want to ensure you are aware that thiazide diuretics are contraindicated for your condition.
D) If you experience any rash or sensitivity to sunlight, let me know immediately.

Correct Answer: A) Be sure to eat potassium-rich foods like bananas.

And B) It's essential to monitor your blood pressure daily, especially since you're taking hydrochlorothiazide.

Explanation of Options:

A) Be sure to eat potassium-rich foods like bananas.

- Why it's right: Thiazide diuretics like hydrochlorothiazide typically cause hypokalemia (low potassium levels). While it's good to encourage a balanced diet, the emphasis should be on potassium supplementation or monitoring potassium intake to prevent hypokalemia.

B) It's essential to monitor your blood pressure daily, especially since you're taking hydrochlorothiazide.

- Why it's right: Monitoring blood pressure is crucial for patients on antihypertensive medications, including hydrochlorothiazide, to ensure effective management of hypertension and assess the medication's efficacy.

C) Since you have chronic kidney disease, I want to ensure you are aware that thiazide diuretics are contraindicated for your condition.

- Why it's wrong: Thiazide diuretics are not outright contraindicated in chronic kidney disease; they can be used in patients with mild to moderate CKD (e.g., stage 2) to manage hypertension. However, they may be less effective as kidney function declines, and careful monitoring is necessary.

D) If you experience any rash or sensitivity to sunlight, let me know immediately.

- Why it's wrong: While it is important for patients to report rashes or photosensitivity as these can be side effects of thiazide diuretics, this statement does not directly address the critical aspects of her treatment and monitoring for effectiveness of the medication. Additionally, other statements are more relevant to her current medication regimen and its effects.

Que: Mrs. Ranjan is a 35-year-old pregnant woman who has been diagnosed with pregnancy-induced hypertension. Her healthcare provider has prescribed a loop diuretic, furosemide, to help control her blood pressure. Mrs. Ranjan has been taking the medication as directed, but she has noticed that she has been feeling very dizzy and lightheaded whenever she stands up. She has also noticed that her urine is a darker color than usual and she is experiencing muscle cramps.

Which of the following is a potential side effect of loop diuretics like furosemide?

a) Hyperkalemia

b) Hypocalcemia

c) Metabolic acidosis

d) Hypovolemia

Answer:

d) Hypovolemia

Explanation: sxLoop diuretics like furosemide are known for their potent diuretic effect, which can lead to excessive fluid and electrolyte loss. Hypovolemia, or a decrease in blood volume, can result from the fluid loss caused by loop diuretics. This can lead to symptoms like dizziness, lightheadedness, dark-colored urine, and muscle cramps. Patients taking loop diuretics should be monitored for signs of electrolyte imbalances and dehydration.

Que : A pregnant woman has been diagnosed with pregnancy-induced hypertension and is prescribed a diuretic to help manage her blood pressure. The healthcare provider prescribes furosemide, a loop diuretic. The patient takes the medication as prescribed and experiences an increase in urine output, but also notices some ringing in her ears and a decrease in her potassium levels.

Which of the following side effects of loop diuretics could the patient be experiencing?
A) Hyponatremia
B) Hypokalemia
C) Dehydration
D) Ototoxicity

To solve this question , we need to review the information provided about loop diuretics and their potential side effects.

Explanation:
Ototoxicity is a known side effect of loop diuretics, specifically furosemide, and can cause ringing in the ears and hearing loss. Loop diuretics can also cause electrolyte imbalances, such as hyponatremia and hypokalemia, as well as dehydration due to the increased urine output. It is important for healthcare providers to monitor patients taking loop diuretics for these potential side effects and make adjustments to the treatment plan as needed.

Patient Profile:
- **Name:** Mr. Thompson
- **Age:** 55
- **Medical History:** Hypertension, heart failure, and type 2 diabetes
- **Current Medications:** Furosemide (a loop diuretic), lisinopril, metformin

Clinical Scenario: Mr. Thompson visits the clinic for a follow-up regarding his heart failure management. He has been experiencing increased fatigue and mild swelling in his legs. The nurse reviews his medication regimen and discusses his symptoms and dietary habits.

Nurse's Statements:
1. "Furosemide will help remove excess fluid, but you should monitor your weight daily to detect any sudden changes."
2. "It's important to avoid foods high in potassium since furosemide can cause potassium loss."
3. "If you notice any ringing in your ears or changes in your hearing, please contact me right away."
4. "Since you have diabetes, it's essential to monitor your blood glucose levels frequently while on furosemide."

Multiple Choice Question
Which statement made by the nurse is correct regarding Mr. Thompson's treatment with furosemide?

A) It's important to avoid foods high in potassium since furosemide can cause potassium loss.
B) If you notice any ringing in your ears or changes in your hearing, please contact me right away.
C) Furosemide will help remove excess fluid, but you should monitor your weight daily to detect any sudden changes.
D) Since you have diabetes, it's essential to monitor your blood glucose levels frequently while on furosemide.

Correct Answer: C) Furosemide will help remove excess fluid, but you should monitor your weight daily to detect any sudden changes.

Explanation of Options:

A) It's important to avoid foods high in potassium since furosemide can cause potassium loss.
- **Why it's wrong:** This statement is incorrect because furosemide is a loop diuretic that can lead to hypokalemia (low potassium levels). Instead, patients are often encouraged to consume potassium-rich foods or take potassium supplements, if necessary, to prevent hypokalemia.

B) If you notice any ringing in your ears or changes in your hearing, please contact me right away.
- **Why it's wrong:** While this statement is partially true, it is less directly relevant than option C. Ototoxicity can occur with furosemide, especially with rapid intravenous administration, so the nurse should be monitoring Mr. Thompson closely, but the focus should also be on fluid management and weight monitoring.

C) Furosemide will help remove excess fluid, but you should monitor your weight daily to detect any sudden changes.
- **Why it's right:** This statement is correct and essential for patients on loop diuretics like furosemide. Monitoring weight daily helps assess fluid retention and the effectiveness of the diuretic therapy, allowing for timely interventions if significant weight changes occur.

D) Since you have diabetes, it's essential to monitor your blood glucose levels frequently while on furosemide.
- **Why it's wrong:** While patients with diabetes should monitor their blood glucose levels, furosemide is not known to significantly affect glucose levels. Therefore, the urgency or emphasis on blood glucose monitoring while specifically taking furosemide is not as critical compared to monitoring weight and electrolytes.

Tuberculosis Medications

Practice Session

Que : Anita, a 35-year-old woman, has been diagnosed with active tuberculosis (TB). She has started treatment with a combination of TB medications and is currently under the care of a nurse. Anita is concerned about her condition and has questions about her treatment plan.

Which TB medication is typically considered first-line treatment for active TB, and what is the primary mode of transmission for TB?

A) Isoniazid; Mode of transmission: Ingestion of contaminated food

B) Rifampin; Mode of transmission: Sexual contact

C) Ethambutol; Mode of transmission: Skin-to-skin contact

D) Pyrazinamide; Mode of transmission: Ingestion of contaminated water

E) Streptomycin; Mode of transmission: Airborne respiratory droplets

F) Levofloxacin; Mode of transmission: Vector-borne through mosquitoes

The first-line treatment for active tuberculosis (TB) typically involves a combination of four key medications: Isoniazid, Rifampin (Rifampicin), Ethambutol, and Pyrazinamide. These drugs work together to effectively combat the TB bacteria and reduce the risk of developing drug-resistant strains. The primary mode of transmission for TB is through airborne respiratory droplets. When an individual with active TB coughs, sneezes, or talks, tiny droplets containing the bacteria are released into the air. These droplets can then be inhaled by others, leading to the spread of the infection.

Option E is correct because airborne respiratory droplets are the primary mode of transmission for TB. Understanding the mode of transmission is crucial for infection control and prevention. Other options are incorrect as primary mode of transmission is incorrect.

Que : A 35-year-old pregnant patient from a high TB burden country has been diagnosed with active tuberculosis. She is prescribed a combination of TB medications as part of her treatment plan. The nurse is responsible for ensuring the patient's safety and adherence to the treatment regimen while considering her pregnancy and cultural background.

Which of the following habit of the patient should the nurse be particularly attentive to in this case?

A) Adherence to the medication schedule

B) Monitoring for drug-induced neuropathy

C) Assessing for drug allergies

D) Implementing isolation precautions

E) Understanding cultural beliefs and practices

F) Involving family or support systems

G) Educating the patient about TB medication

H) Avoiding streptomycin and suggesting ethambutol as an alternative

Explanation:

Correct Answers: A) Adherence to the medication schedule is crucial in this case because the patient is pregnant, and untreated TB can pose serious risks to both the mother and the fetus. Ensuring that the patient takes the prescribed medications as scheduled is essential for effective treatment. H) Avoiding streptomycin and suggesting ethambutol as an alternative is also important because streptomycin is contraindicated during pregnancy due to its potential to cause harm to the developing fetus. Ethambutol is a safer alternative for pregnant patients.

Explanation for Incorrect Options:

B) Monitoring for drug-induced neuropathy: While monitoring for drug-induced neuropathy is important, it is not specific to the pregnant patient population and is a consideration for all TB patients.

C) Assessing for drug allergies: While assessing for drug allergies is a critical nursing responsibility, it is not specific to pregnant patients and should be done for all TB patients.

D) Implementing isolation precautions: Isolation precautions are important to prevent the spread of TB but are not specific to pregnant patients. They apply to all patients with active TB.

E) Understanding cultural beliefs and practices: While understanding cultural considerations is important for providing culturally competent care, it is not directly related to the specific needs of a pregnant TB patient.

F) Involving family or support systems: Involving family or support systems is a good strategy for improving adherence but is not unique to pregnant TB patients.

G) Educating the patient about TB medication: Educating the patient about TB medication is important but does not specifically address the unique needs of a pregnant TB patient who should avoid certain medications like streptomycin.

Que: A 7-year-old boy named David presents to the clinic with a persistent cough, fever, and weight loss. His mother reports that David has been feeling fatigued and has not been eating well. David's family has a history of tuberculosis, as his older brother was recently diagnosed with active tuberculosis. The healthcare provider decides to conduct a tuberculin skin test (TST) to assess David's risk of tuberculosis infection.

What is the most critical factor contributing to the emergence of multidrug-resistant strains of *M. tuberculosis* in David's case?

A. Family history of tuberculosis.

B. Noncompliance with treatment by family members.

C. Geographic location of the family residence.

D. Presence of symptoms such as cough and fever.

Correct Answer:

B. Noncompliance with treatment by family members.

Explanation of Options

- **A. Family history of tuberculosis.**
  Wrong. While a family history may indicate a higher risk of exposure, it does not directly cause multidrug resistance. Resistance is more closely linked to treatment adherence.

- **B. Noncompliance with treatment by family members.**
  Right. Noncompliance with prescribed treatment regimens in the family, especially in individuals diagnosed with active tuberculosis, can lead to inadequate control of the infection, resulting in the development of drug-resistant strains.

- **C. Geographic location of the family residence.**
  Wrong. Although living in urban low-income areas may increase exposure to tuberculosis, it is the noncompliance with treatment that primarily contributes to drug resistance.

- **D. Presence of symptoms such as cough and fever.**
  Wrong. While symptoms indicate potential infection, they are not a direct factor in the development of multidrug-resistant strains. Symptoms reflect the disease's activity rather than its resistance profile.

Integumentary system / Drugs

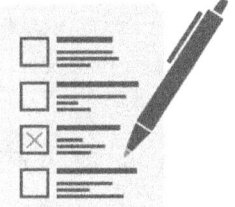

Practice Session

Que: Mr. Johnson is a 40-year-old man who suffered third-degree burns on his chest and back in a workplace accident. His healthcare provider prescribes daily wound dressing changes using a hydrogel dressing. After a few days of treatment, Mr. Johnson complains of a foul odor emanating from his burns and notices an increase in the wound's drainage.

What should the nurse do in response to Mr. Johnson's symptoms?

A) Continue with the hydrogel dressing changes as prescribed.

B) Switch to a silver-impregnated dressing for daily changes.

C) Clean the burn wounds thoroughly with a mild antiseptic solution and continue with hydrogel dressing changes.

D) Consult the healthcare provider for a possible infection and appropriate wound care adjustments.

Correct answer: D

Rationale: The correct course of action in response to Mr. Johnson's symptoms is to consult the healthcare provider for a possible infection and appropriate wound care adjustments. Option A is incorrect because continuing with the hydrogel dressing without addressing the foul odor and increased drainage may lead to complications. Option B may not be necessary if there's no sign of infection. Option C is not sufficient to address the potential infection and may need medical evaluation.

Que: A patient presents to the emergency department with a chemical burn injury on their lower leg. The burn covers an area of 4 inches in diameter and appears to be a partial-thickness burn. The patient reports intense pain and blistering at the burn site. The burn occurred when the patient accidentally spilled a corrosive chemical on their leg.

What is the size of the burn on the patient's leg according to the "rule of nines?"

A. 4%

B. 9%

C. 18%

D. 36%

Correct answer: A (4%)

The "rule of nines" is a method used to estimate the total body surface area (TBSA) affected by burns. According to this rule:

The total body surface area of an adult is divided into sections, each representing approximately 9% or a multiple of 9%.

The front and back of each leg represent 18% of the total body surface area (9% for the front and 9% for the back).

Since the burn is on the lower leg, which represents 9% of the body surface area, you need to calculate the percentage of this area covered by the burn.

Given that the burn covers an area of 4 inches in diameter, and this diameter is a small part of the entire lower leg area, the burn's coverage is less than the whole lower leg surface. Therefore, if you estimate it conservatively, the coverage of a 4-inch diameter area would be roughly a small percentage of the 9% for the leg.

Given the options provided and considering the relative size of the burn area compared to the whole leg, the most accurate choice is:

A) 4%

This is a reasonable estimate for a burn area of that size on the lower leg, which represents a small portion of the total 9% surface area for that leg.

Que: A 28-year-old female patient has sustained a burn injury on her chest and abdomen. The burn is a full-thickness burn, characterized by a dry, white, and leathery appearance. The burn covers 20% of the patient's body surface area, with the majority of the burn located on her chest and abdomen. The patient is in significant pain and exhibits signs of hypovolemic shock.

Which of the following is the most appropriate fluid resuscitation formula for this patient?

A) Modified Brooke

B) Parkland

C) Modified Parkland

D) Hypertonic saline

Correct answer:

B) Parkland

Rationale: Parkland formula is the most appropriate fluid resuscitation formula for this patient because it is designed for burns involving a significant surface area. The Parkland formula involves the administration of lactated Ringer's solution, typically in the first 24 hours, to manage hypovolemia and provide the necessary fluid replacement. It is recommended for full-thickness burns as well. Modified

Brooke is primarily intended for deep partial-thickness burns and may not be the best choice in this case. Modified Parkland is a variation of the Parkland formula and is typically used in cases where the burn occurred longer than 24 hours ago. Hypertonic saline is not the first-line choice for fluid resuscitation in burn patients.

Que: Sanjeeta is a 23-year-old woman who has been suffering from severe acne for several years. She has tried a variety of over-the-counter products and topical medications, but nothing seems to be helping. She decides to visit a dermatologist for further treatment. The dermatologist diagnoses her with severe acne and prescribes isotretinoin as the recommended treatment. Sanjeeta is hesitant to take the medication because she has heard about the potential side effects, including bone marrow depression and ulcerative colitis.

Which of the following is the most effective treatment option for severe acne?

a) Gentle cleansing

b) Topical antimicrobials

c) Oral antibiotics

d) Isotretinoin

Answer: d) Isotretinoin

Rationale:

>Isotretinoin is the recommended treatment option for severe acne. The other options listed (gentle cleansing, topical antimicrobials, and oral antibiotics) are all taken as treatment options for mild or moderate acne. Therefore, option d) Isotretinoin is the most effective treatment option for severe acne.
>Isotretinoin is a medication that is specifically designed to treat severe acne. It works by reducing the production of oil in the skin, which can help to prevent the formation of new acne lesions. It is generally considered to be the most effective treatment option for severe acne because it can help to clear up the skin quickly and prevent new breakouts from occurring. Other treatment options, such as gentle cleansing and topical antimicrobials, may not be as effective for severe acne because they do not address the underlying causes of the condition.

Antifungal Medications

> **Understanding antifungal medications is essential for effective treatment of fungal infections. It involves recognizing various classes like azoles, polyenes, echinocandins, and allylamines, each with distinct mechanisms of action. For example, fluconazole, an azole antifungal, inhibits fungal cytochrome P450 enzymes, making it effective against fungal infections. Identifying indications for specific medications is crucial; for severe systemic fungal infections like invasive candidiasis, echinocandins such as caspofungin are preferred. Patient-specific factors, including age and comorbidities, guide treatment decisions. Adjusting amphotericin B dosage for elderly patients with renal impairment prevents nephrotoxicity. Vigilance for common side effects, such as visual disturbances with voriconazole, ensures timely intervention. Understanding drug interactions, like the increased bleeding risk when combining warfarin with fluconazole, prevents complications. Safety measures, including patient education on oral nystatin suspension administration, promote effective treatment. Regular monitoring for adverse effects, such as electrolyte imbalances with furosemide therapy, enhances patient safety. Staying informed about resistance patterns and choosing appropriate agents, like echinocandins in regions with fluconazole-resistant Candida glabrata, optimizes treatment efficacy. Recognizing allergic reactions and promptly discontinuing terbinafine if a diffuse rash occurs prevents worsening reactions. Considering pregnancy and lactation, topical treatments like miconazole are preferred to minimize systemic drug exposure. Determining the duration of therapy based on infection type ensures comprehensive treatment. Tailoring antifungal therapy to local resistance profiles maximizes treatment success and patient outcomes.**

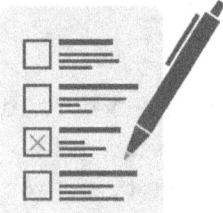

Practice Session

Que : A 72-year-old male patient with a history of chronic obstructive pulmonary disease (COPD) and type 2 diabetes is admitted to the hospital with a severe fungal lung infection. The patient is prescribed antifungal medication as part of the treatment plan.

Which of the following statements by the nurse is correct based on the given case study?

A) The patient should be given oral nystatin suspension for treatment.

B) Fluconazole, an azole antifungal, is the most suitable choice for this patient.

C) Amphotericin B should be administered without any dosage adjustments.

D) There is no need to monitor the patient for adverse effects of antifungal medications.

Explanation of Options:

A) Incorrect. Oral nystatin suspension is typically used for oral thrush, not for severe fungal lung infections like the one described in the case study.

B) Correct. Fluconazole is an azole antifungal medication that can be used for severe fungal infections, especially if the patient has comorbidities like COPD and diabetes. It inhibits fungal cytochrome P450 enzymes and is a suitable choice.

C) Incorrect. Amphotericin B is known for its nephrotoxicity and often requires dosage adjustments, especially in elderly patients and those with renal impairment. The patient in this case has both age and comorbidities that should be considered.

D) Incorrect. It is essential to monitor patients for adverse effects when they are on antifungal medications, as these drugs can have various side effects. Monitoring helps ensure patient safety and effective treatment.

Correct Answer: B (Fluconazole, an azole antifungal, is the most suitable choice for this patient.)

Que : A 65-year-old male patient with a history of leukemia has been admitted to the oncology unit for chemotherapy. During his hospital stay, he develops a fever and a persistent cough. The nursing staff decides to initiate empirical antifungal therapy with voriconazole due to the patient's neutropenic status and the presence of fever.

Which of the following statements regarding the patient's antifungal therapy is correct?

A) The choice of voriconazole for empirical therapy is appropriate, and no further evaluation is needed.

B) The patient's renal function should be monitored, as dose adjustments may be necessary for voriconazole.

C) Patient compliance barriers should be addressed to ensure treatment adherence.

D) Fungal cultures and sensitivity testing should be obtained to guide antifungal therapy.

Explanation: A) Incorrect. While the initiation of empirical antifungal therapy with voriconazole is a valid approach in neutropenic patients with fever, this statement does not address any potential dose adjustments or monitoring requirements.

B) Correct. This statement is correct. Patients receiving voriconazole should have their renal function monitored because dose adjustments may be necessary to prevent adverse effects, including nephrotoxicity.

C) Incorrect. While addressing patient compliance barriers is essential, this statement does not directly pertain to the choice of antifungal therapy or the need for dose adjustments in this scenario.

D) Incorrect. While obtaining fungal cultures and sensitivity testing is generally important in guiding antifungal therapy, in the context of empirical therapy, the goal is to initiate treatment promptly without waiting for culture results.

Therefore, option B is the correct answer because it addresses the specific need to monitor renal function and consider dose adjustments when using voriconazole for empirical antifungal therapy in a neutropenic patient.

Que: A 35-year-old female patient with a history of cryptococcal meningitis is admitted to the hospital for treatment with amphotericin B. The nurse prepares to administer the medication intravenously.

Which of the following nursing actions is most important to implement prior to administering amphotericin B?

A. "Ensure the patient has been fasting for at least 8 hours before administration."
B. "Administer an antihistamine to the patient to prevent infusion reactions."
C. "Dilute the medication in saline solution for better solubility."
D. "Infuse the medication rapidly to reduce treatment time."

Correct Answer: B

Explanation of Each Option:

- **Option A: Incorrect**
    - Fasting is not a requirement for administering amphotericin B. Unlike some medications that must be taken on an empty stomach, amphotericin B is administered intravenously, so dietary restrictions are not necessary.

- **Option B: Correct**
    - Administering an antihistamine (along with antipyretics or corticosteroids) is a critical nursing action to help prevent potential infusion-related reactions, which can occur with amphotericin B administration.

- **Option C: Incorrect**
    - Amphotericin B should be diluted in dextrose solution, not saline, as saline can precipitate the drug. This is essential to ensure safe and effective administration.

- **Option D: Incorrect**
    - Infusing amphotericin B rapidly is not advisable; it should be infused slowly over 2-6 hours to minimize the risk of infusion-related reactions, such as fever, chills, and hypotension. Proper administration rate is critical for patient safety.

Que: A 50-year-old male patient diagnosed with histoplasmosis is prescribed itraconazole. The nurse is preparing to educate the patient about the medication and its administration.

Which of the following statements made by the nurse regarding the administration of itraconazole is most accurate?

A. "You can take the capsules with any type of beverage to aid swallowing."
B. "It's best to take the oral solution on an empty stomach for optimal absorption."
C. "You should take the capsules with a full meal to enhance absorption."
D. "You can take the medication at any time of the day, as it does not affect absorption."

Correct Answer: C

Explanation of Each Option:

- **Option A: Incorrect**
    - The capsules should not be taken with just any beverage. They must be taken with a full meal to improve absorption, particularly because certain foods can enhance the drug's bioavailability.

- **Option B: Incorrect**
    - While the oral solution should be taken on an empty stomach for optimal absorption, this statement does not apply to the capsules, which require a full meal. Therefore, this option is not accurate in the context of educating the patient about itraconazole capsules.

- **Option C: Correct**
    - This statement is accurate. Itraconazole capsules should be taken with a full meal to enhance their absorption, making this the correct response.

- **Option D: Incorrect**
    - Timing is important for itraconazole absorption. The capsules must be taken with food, and taking the medication at any time of the day without regard for meals can lead to decreased efficacy. Thus, this statement is misleading.

Que: A 45-year-old female patient is being treated for candidiasis with fluconazole. The nurse is reviewing the patient's lab results and is preparing to provide education regarding the medication. Which of the following statements regarding fluconazole administration should the nurse emphasize to the patient?

A. "Fluconazole can be taken with any type of beverage, including fruit juices."
B. "You should take this medication only if you experience symptoms of infection."
C. "It's important to inform your healthcare provider if you have any kidney problems."
D. "Fluconazole should be taken at least one hour before meals for best absorption."

Correct Answer: C

Explanation of Each Option:

- **Option A: Incorrect**

- While fluconazole can be taken with some beverages, certain drinks like fruit juices might affect its absorption or efficacy. It's best to take the medication with water, but this option does not provide a comprehensive guideline.

- **Option B: Incorrect**
    - This statement is misleading. Fluconazole should be taken as prescribed by the healthcare provider, not only when symptoms are present. Patients must adhere to the treatment plan to effectively clear the infection and prevent relapse.

- **Option C: Correct**
    - This statement is accurate and important. The nurse should emphasize to the patient that they need to inform their healthcare provider of any kidney problems, as fluconazole is metabolized by the liver and excreted by the kidneys, and renal impairment may necessitate a dosage adjustment.

- **Option D: Incorrect**
    - This statement is not accurate. Fluconazole can be taken with or without food, and there is no strict requirement to take it at least one hour before meals for optimal absorption. Therefore, this option does not accurately reflect the administration guidelines for fluconazole.

Narcotic Antagonists

Practice Session

Que: A 28-year-old male presents to the emergency department after being found unconscious due to a suspected opioid overdose.

Which of the following statements correctly describes the appropriate use of naloxone in this scenario?

A. "Naloxone can be administered orally for the fastest effect."

B. "Naloxone should only be used if the patient has been unresponsive for more than 10 minutes."

C. "Naloxone can reverse the effects of an opioid overdose within minutes when given by injection or nasal spray."

D. "Naloxone should be administered only after checking for a pulse."

E. "Naloxone is used to enhance the effects of opioids in overdose cases."

Correct Answer: C

Explanation:

Option A: Incorrect

Naloxone is not administered orally for rapid reversal; it is typically given via injection or nasal spray for quick action in emergency situations.

Option B: Incorrect

Naloxone should be used as soon as an opioid overdose is suspected, regardless of how long the patient has been unresponsive. Delaying treatment could lead to severe complications or death.

Option C: Correct

This statement accurately describes naloxone's use. It can reverse opioid overdose effects rapidly when administered by injection or nasal spray, making it an essential emergency intervention.

Option D: Incorrect

Checking for a pulse is not a prerequisite for administering naloxone. The focus should be on recognizing signs of opioid overdose, such as unresponsiveness or respiratory depression.

Option E: Incorrect

Naloxone is not used to enhance opioid effects; rather, it works by blocking the effects of opioids to reverse overdose symptoms.

Que : When should a nurse administer a narcotic antagonist to a patient?

A) As a preventive measure to avoid opioid addiction.

B) In cases of severe anxiety or panic attacks.

C) In cases of opioid overdose or respiratory depression following opioid administration.

D) During routine pain management for chronic conditions.

Explanation:

Correct Answer: C) In cases of opioid overdose or respiratory depression following opioid administration.

Explanation: Narcotic antagonists, such as naloxone, are administered in cases of opioid overdose or when a patient experiences respiratory depression due to the effects of opioids. These medications are used as an emergency intervention to reverse the life-threatening effects of opioids and restore normal breathing. Options A, B, and D do not represent appropriate situations for administering narcotic antagonists.

Que: Which of the following statements accurately reflects the key considerations for administering naloxone in this situation?

A. "Naloxone can be given orally for the quickest effect in an overdose situation."
B. "It is important to monitor the patient for withdrawal symptoms after administering naloxone."
C. "Naloxone should be given only once, as repeated doses can cause complications."
D. "Naloxone is not effective if administered as a nasal spray."
E. "Naloxone is only used in hospital settings and is not needed at home."

Correct Answer: B

Explanation:

- **Option A: Incorrect**
    - Naloxone should not be administered orally in overdose situations, as it is not effective that way. It is given via injection or as a nasal spray for rapid action.

- **Option B: Correct**
    - Monitoring for withdrawal symptoms is crucial after administering naloxone, especially if the patient is dependent on opioids. While these symptoms can be uncomfortable, they are not life-threatening.

- **Option C: Incorrect**

- o Naloxone may need to be given in repeated doses depending on the severity of the overdose and the patient's response to the initial dose. Limiting it to only one dose may not adequately address the overdose.

- **Option D: Incorrect**
  - o Naloxone is effective when administered as a nasal spray. This route of administration provides a quick and convenient method for reversing opioid overdose.

- **Option E: Incorrect**
  - o Naloxone is essential not only in hospital settings but also for use at home, especially for individuals at risk of opioid overdose. Increasing access to naloxone is critical for saving lives.

Anticancer

Cytotoxic Chemotherapy:

These drugs work by damaging or killing rapidly dividing cancer cells.

Common drugs include cisplatin, cyclophosphamide, and paclitaxel.

Side effects: Nausea, vomiting, bone marrow suppression (low blood cell counts), hair loss.

Targeted Therapy:

Target specific molecules or pathways involved in cancer growth.

Examples are imatinib (Gleevec) and trastuzumab (Herceptin).

Side effects: May target normal cells, leading to skin rash, diarrhea, cardiac issues.

Hormone Therapy:

Block hormones like estrogen in hormone-sensitive cancers (e.g., breast, prostate).

Tamoxifen and leuprolide are common examples.

Side effects: Hormonal imbalances, hot flashes, bone density loss.

Immunotherapy:

Boost the body's immune system to fight cancer.

Drugs like pembrolizumab (Keytruda) and nivolumab (Opdivo).

Side effects: Immune-related adverse events (irAEs) like colitis, pneumonitis.

Easy Tips for Remembering:

Cytotoxic Chemotherapy can be remembered as "Killing Cells" - they kill rapidly dividing cells.

Targeted Therapy is like a "Targeted Missile" - precise treatment targeting specific molecules.

Hormone Therapy is related to hormones; think "Hormone Blockers."

Immunotherapy is like "Boosting the Immune System" - it helps the immune system fight cancer.

Important Notes on Side Effects:

"Cytotoxic" sounds like "sick-toxic." These drugs make you feel sick with side effects.

"Targeted" therapy is precise but can also target normal cells, causing issues.

"Hormone" therapy often leads to hormonal imbalances.

"Immuno"therapy can result in immune-related adverse events (irAEs).

Drug Interactions:

Check for interactions with other medications as some anticancer drugs can affect liver enzymes (e.g., cytochrome P450) and impact the metabolism of other drugs.

Antacids, for example, can reduce the absorption of some oral anticancer drugs.

Always review the patient's medication list for potential interactions.

Que: Which of the following statements of the nurse indicates appropriate client education for a patient undergoing radiation therapy?

A. "Make sure to use powder or lotion on the irradiated area to soothe the skin after washing."
B. "It's best to use a washcloth to scrub the area thoroughly during your daily bath."
C. "Try to keep the markings on your skin intact, as they help guide the radiation treatment."
D. "After radiation therapy, you should wear tight clothing to protect the treated area from external elements."
E. "Avoid exposing the treated area to direct sunlight or heat to prevent further skin irritation."

Correct Answers: C and E

Explanation:

- **Option A: Incorrect**
    - Using powders, ointments, lotions, or creams on the irradiated area is not advised unless prescribed by the radiologist. These products can irritate the sensitive skin, potentially affecting the effectiveness of the radiation treatment.

- **Option B: Incorrect**
    - Using a washcloth and scrubbing can irritate the skin in the irradiated area. It's recommended to wash the area gently with the hand to avoid causing irritation or damage to the sensitive skin.

- **Option C: Correct**
    - Keeping the skin markings intact is crucial as they guide where the radiation needs to be focused. Removing them can affect the accuracy of the radiation therapy.

- **Option D: Incorrect**

- o   Wearing tight clothing over the treated area can rub or irritate the skin, leading to discomfort or skin damage. It is advisable to wear soft, loose-fitting clothing.

- **Option E: Correct**

  - o   Avoiding direct sunlight or heat exposure to the irradiated area is important, as these can exacerbate skin irritation or cause burns, worsening skin reactions during radiation therapy.

Case Study: A nurse is caring for a patient undergoing brachytherapy for cervical cancer. The patient's family arrives, including a pregnant daughter and a 10-year-old child.

Multiple Choice Question: Which of the following statements of the nurse indicates proper understanding of the safety guidelines when caring for a patient with sealed radiation implants?

A. "The patient's family can visit freely as long as they don't stay too long."
B. "Visitors must stay at least 6 feet away from the patient and should limit their visits to 30 minutes."
C. "It's okay for the patient's pregnant daughter to visit, but she should wear a protective apron."
D. "The 10-year-old child can visit as long as he stays at a distance."
E. "No pregnant women or children under 16 should be allowed to visit the patient."

Correct Answers: B and E

Explanation:

- **Option A: Incorrect**

  - o   Visitors cannot visit freely; strict limitations are in place to minimize radiation exposure. They must follow specific guidelines for time and distance.

- **Option B: Correct**

  - o   Visitors should limit their visits to 30 minutes per day and stay at least 6 feet away from the patient to minimize exposure, which aligns with safety protocols.

- **Option C: Incorrect**

  - o   Pregnant women are not allowed to visit patients with sealed radiation implants, regardless of protective measures, due to the risk of radiation exposure.

- **Option D: Incorrect**

  - o   Children under 16 should not visit patients undergoing brachytherapy, as they are at increased risk of radiation exposure.

- **Option E: Correct**

  - o   The guideline explicitly states that pregnant women and children under 16 should not visit patients with sealed radiation implants to ensure their safety.

Que : You are a nurse working in an oncology unit, and you are responsible for caring for a patient named Anita, who is undergoing chemotherapy for breast cancer. Anita is receiving a combination of chemotherapy agents as part of her treatment plan. The primary healthcare provider has instructed you to closely monitor Anita for potential side effects and adverse reactions to the anticancer medications.

One day, while administering Anita's chemotherapy, you notice that she suddenly becomes very anxious and begins complaining of difficulty breathing and chest pain. You quickly assess her vital signs and find that her heart rate has increased significantly, her blood pressure has dropped, and she is developing hives on her skin. Anita's caretaker is present and expresses concern about her condition.

Which of the following best describes the situation, and what actions should the nurse take based on the given strategies for managing anticancer medications?

A) Anita is experiencing a common side effect of chemotherapy, and the nurse should reassure her and continue the infusion.

B) Anita is having a typical reaction to chemotherapy, and the nurse should administer an antihistamine.

C) Anita is likely experiencing an anaphylactic reaction to the chemotherapy, and the nurse should stop the infusion immediately and administer epinephrine and call for emergency assistance.

D) Anita's anxiety is unrelated to the chemotherapy, and the nurse should offer emotional support.

E) Anita is experiencing a mild allergic reaction to the chemotherapy, and the nurse should continue the infusion but monitor her closely.

F) Anita is having a common side effect of chemotherapy, and the nurse should administer a bronchodilator to relieve her breathing difficulties.

Explanation:

C) Anita is likely experiencing an anaphylactic reaction to the chemotherapy, and the nurse should stop the infusion immediately and administer epinephrine and call for emergency assistance.

Explanation:

Option C is correct because it aligns with the "Monitor for Adverse Reactions" strategy. The sudden onset of severe shortness of breath, chest pain, hives, increased heart rate, and decreased blood pressure suggests an anaphylactic reaction, which is a severe and life-threatening adverse reaction to the chemotherapy. The nurse should take immediate action by stopping the infusion, administering epinephrine to reverse the allergic reaction, and seeking emergency assistance.

Option E is partially correct because it recognizes that Anita is experiencing an allergic reaction. However, it is not appropriate to continue the infusion without addressing the allergic reaction. Monitoring is important, but in the presence of an allergic reaction, it is essential to stop the infusion and provide appropriate intervention.

Palliative Care Principles

Strategy: Understand the role of palliative care in cancer treatment and its focus on symptom management and improving the patient's quality of life.

Example: A question may inquire about the nurse's actions when a patient with advanced cancer experiences severe pain. Knowing to prioritize pain control and consider opioids for pain management aligns with palliative care principles.

Chemotherapy Regimens:

Strategy: Familiarize yourself with common chemotherapy regimens and their indications for various types and stages of cancer.

Example: You might encounter a question about the appropriate chemotherapy regimen for a patient with stage III breast cancer, testing your knowledge of treatment protocols like AC (doxorubicin and cyclophosphamide) followed by Taxol.

Nutritional Support:

Strategy: Recognize the importance of nutritional support in cancer care, especially when patients experience appetite loss or weight changes.

Example: You may be asked about interventions for a patient receiving chemotherapy who is struggling with poor appetite. Advising small, frequent, nutrient-rich meals and considering antiemetic medications can be a relevant response.

Chemotherapy-Induced Peripheral Neuropathy (CIPN):

Strategy: Be aware of CIPN as a potential side effect of some chemotherapy drugs and understand its assessment and management.

Example: A question could involve a patient reporting numbness and tingling in their extremities after receiving chemotherapy. Recognizing these symptoms as CIPN and advising measures to minimize further nerve damage can be essential.

Rescue Medications:

Strategy: Learn about rescue medications used to counteract specific side effects of anticancer treatments, such as colony-stimulating factors for neutropenia.

Example: You might be asked about the administration of filgrastim (Neupogen) to a patient undergoing chemotherapy. Understanding when to administer this medication to boost white blood cell production can be crucial.

Psychosocial Support:

Strategy: Acknowledge the emotional and psychological impact of cancer diagnosis and treatment on patients and their families.

Example: A question may focus on providing emotional support to a newly diagnosed cancer patient. Identifying the need for counseling resources or support groups and offering them to the patient can be a relevant response.

Patient Information: Mr. Smith, a 65-year-old gentleman, has been diagnosed with advanced-stage lung cancer. He is currently receiving palliative care to manage his symptoms and improve his quality of life. As a nurse caring for Mr. Smith, it's essential to adhere to palliative care principles.

MCQ Que : What is the primary focus of palliative care for patients like Mr. Smith with advanced cancer?

A) Aggressive cancer treatment to achieve remission.

B) Symptom management and improving quality of life.

C) Psychological counseling for the patient's family.

D) Nutritional support to boost the patient's appetite.

Explanation: B) Symptom management and improving quality of life.

Option A (Aggressive cancer treatment to achieve remission): This option is incorrect because palliative care in advanced cancer aims to relieve symptoms and improve the patient's comfort and quality of life. It does not involve aggressive treatments with the intent of achieving remission, which is typically pursued in curative care.

Option C (Psychological counseling for the patient's family): This option is incorrect because while psychosocial support is an important aspect of cancer care, the primary focus of palliative care is on the patient's well-being, comfort, and symptom management. Psychological counseling for the patient's family may be part of comprehensive palliative care but is not the primary focus.

Option D (Nutritional support to boost the patient's appetite): This option is incorrect because while nutritional support is essential in cancer care, it is not the primary focus of palliative care. Palliative care primarily addresses symptom management, pain control, and improving the patient's overall quality of life. Nutritional support may be included in the care plan, but it is not the primary goal.

Option B (Symptom management and improving quality of life): This is the correct answer. Palliative care for patients with advanced cancer, like Mr. Smith, focuses on symptom management to provide relief from pain, discomfort, and other distressing symptoms. The primary goal is to enhance the patient's quality of life and ensure their comfort during their illness.

Que: Which of the following statements of the nurse indicates an appropriate understanding of palliative care in cancer treatment?

A. "My primary goal is to cure the patient's cancer completely, regardless of their comfort level."

B. "Pain control is not as important as ensuring the patient adheres to chemotherapy schedules."

C. "I will provide opioids as needed to manage severe pain and enhance the patient's quality of life."

D. "The most important aspect of my care is ensuring strict dietary restrictions for the patient."

E. "I will consider the patient's comfort and quality of life while managing symptoms effectively."

Correct Answers: C and E

Explanation:

Option A: Incorrect

Palliative care's main goal is to enhance the patient's quality of life, not to provide a cure. The statement shows a misunderstanding of the palliative care philosophy, which focuses on comfort and symptom relief rather than curing the disease.

Option B: Incorrect

Pain control is a critical part of palliative care. Prioritizing chemotherapy schedules over managing pain contradicts the principles of palliative care, which emphasize comfort and quality of life.

Option C: Correct

This statement aligns well with palliative care principles, focusing on pain management through the appropriate use of opioids. Managing severe pain is a cornerstone of palliative care for patients with advanced cancer.

Option D: Incorrect

Strict dietary restrictions are not typically a priority in palliative care. Instead, the focus is on providing comfort, which includes encouraging whatever the patient is comfortable eating to maintain strength and quality of life.

Option E: Correct

This statement reflects an understanding that palliative care involves symptom management with an emphasis on the patient's comfort and quality of life, which are central goals of palliative care interventions.

Que: Which of the following statements of the nurse indicates an appropriate approach to managing a patient with congestive heart failure (CHF) in a palliative care setting?

A. "I will focus primarily on fluid restriction and medication adherence to reduce hospital readmissions."
B. "The patient's quality of life is my priority, so I will work with them to manage symptoms such as breathlessness and fatigue."
C. "I will avoid discussing prognosis with the patient to prevent causing anxiety."
D. "It's essential to maintain a strict sodium-restricted diet to slow the progression of heart failure."
E. "I will offer supportive measures, like positioning and oxygen therapy, to alleviate discomfort from dyspnea."

Correct Answers: B and E

Explanation:

- **Option A: Incorrect**
    - While fluid restriction and medication adherence are important in managing CHF, the focus in a palliative care setting is on symptom relief and improving quality of life, rather than just preventing readmissions.

- **Option B: Correct**
    - This statement correctly reflects the principles of palliative care, which prioritize symptom management (e.g., breathlessness and fatigue) and overall quality of life for the patient.

- **Option C: Incorrect**
    - Open communication about prognosis is an essential part of palliative care. Avoiding such discussions may prevent the patient from making informed decisions about their care and end-of-life preferences.

- **Option D: Incorrect**
    - Although sodium restriction can help manage CHF, the rigid application of dietary restrictions is less important in palliative care. The goal is to enhance comfort and quality of life, which may involve balancing dietary needs with the patient's preferences.

- **Option E: Correct**
    - This statement demonstrates a good understanding of symptom management in palliative care. Providing supportive measures like oxygen therapy and positioning can help alleviate the discomfort associated with dyspnea, improving the patient's comfort.

Further Reading : Recommended Resources

Resource Book I:

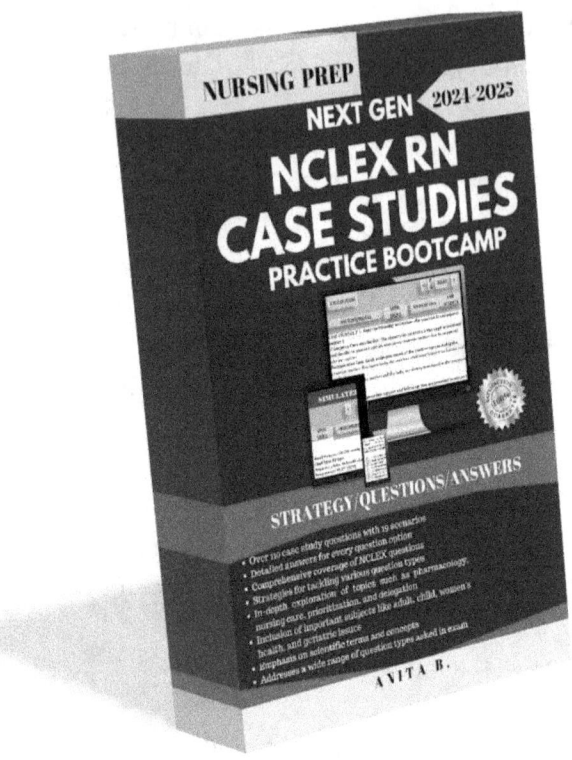

Search in Amazon (Nclex RN Case Studies by Anita B.) or type the following address in your search bar: https://a.co/d/4j0lRQU

- The Natural Fear of Case Studies: Embarking on your NCLEX RN journey may evoke apprehension about case studies. These real-world scenarios require practical application, fueling uncertainty and pressure.
- Conquering the Fear: Case studies are integral to the NCLEX RN exam, shaping competent nurses. Mastering them means honing analytical skills for real-world nursing challenges.
- Bridging Fear to Confidence: The "NCLEX RN Case Studies Exam Practice Bootcamp" offers 100+ case study question, turning fear into familiarity through detailed explanations and strategies.
- Learning from Errors: Understanding why incorrect answers falter is as vital as grasping correct ones. The book ensures valuable insights from both successes and mistakes.

Free Training Awaits !!

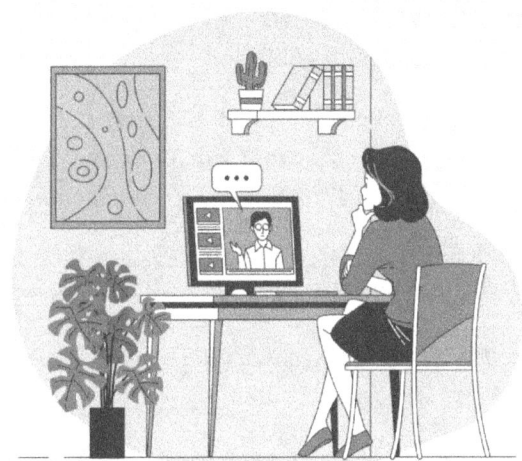

00 : 00 : 00 : 00
DAYS   HOURS   MINUTES   SECONDS

100 STUDENTS SELECTED EACH MONTH !
JOIN THE FREE FASTTRACK NCLEX-RN CRASH COURSE BEFORE THE LINK EXPIRES...
IT'S 100% FREE
SCROLL DOWN FOR DETAILS !!!

First name

Email

Let's Get Started

Not Joined Yet ?

Discover all the tricks revealed in our NCLEX-RN Crash Course! We cover strategies for Next Generation NCLEX exams. From essential NCLEX strategies to questions, basic pharmacology, and care, we've got you covered. Learn how to prepare for the NCLEX in less than 30 days with our comprehensive program. Here are 7 reasons to participate:

Limited availability: Our crash course runs only once per month, so seize the opportunity now!

Free tricks and tips: Gain insights on preparing for different topics and questions in the shortest time possible.

Pharmacology guidance: Master difficult pharmacological and nursing management concepts with expert guidance.

Access to flashcards and quizzes: Reinforce your learning with valuable resources.

Exclusive Facebook group: Join our NCLEX MENTORS community to connect with peers, team members, and coaches.

No recordings available: The value shared in our course is exclusive and live, so don't miss out!

Absolutely free: No charges involved - simply enter your email address, no credit card required. Join now and take charge of your NCLEX preparation journey!

Bibliography

Bhattarai, A. (2023). *New Next Generation NCLEX RN Question Bank 2023/24: BIGBOOK of Question & Answer Practice (NEW NEXT GENERATION NCLEX RN EXAM INTENSIVE PREPARATION SERIES)*. Independently published.

Bhattarai, A., & Subedi, G. (2023). *Mastering New/Next Generation NCLEX RN Pharmacology: Theory, Strategies, and Examples with Case Studies - NEW 2023/24 Guide (NEW ... NCLEX RN EXAM INTENSIVE PREPARATION SERIES)*. Independently published.

Kaplan Nursing. (2015). *NCLEX-RN Drug Guide: 300 Medications You Need to Know for the Exam (Kaplan Test Prep) (Sixth edition)*. Kaplan Publishing.

Lippincott Williams & Wilkins. (2021). *Nursing2022 Drug Handbook (Nursing Drug Handbook) Forty-Second, North American Edition*.

Meloni, S., Medical Creations, & Mastenbjörk, M. (2021). *Pharmacology Review - A Comprehensive Reference Guide for Medical, Nursing, and Paramedic Students*. Medical Creations.

Myers, E. (2021). *MedSurg Notes: Nurse's Clinical Pocket Guide Fifth Edition (5th ed.)*. F.A. Davis Company.

Schull, P. (2013). *McGraw-Hill Nurses Drug Handbook, Seventh Edition (McGraw-Hill's Nurses Drug Handbook) (7th ed.)*. McGraw Hill / Medical.

Silvestri, L. A., & Silvestri, A. (2022). *Saunders comprehensive review for the NCLEX-RN® examination (9th ed.)*. Saunders.

Tucker, R. G. (2021). *2022 Lippincott Pocket Drug Guide for Nurses [Kindle Edition]*. Wolters Kluwer Health. ASIN: B09FFNXSYP.

nclex.com/test-plans.page

Dear Reader,

Thank you for taking the time to read NEW NCLEX RN PRACTICE QUESTION BANK. I hope that you found the information and resources in this book helpful as you prepare for the NCLEX exam.

I am grateful for your support and are committed to helping you achieve your goal of becoming a nurse. If you found this book useful, I would greatly appreciate it if you could share it with others who may also benefit from its content.

Please don't hesitate to reach out to me if you have any questions or feedback. I would love to hear from you and hear about your success on the NCLEX exam.

Once again, thank you for choosing 'NEW NCLEX RN PRACTICE QUESTION BANK and for your continued support of my work.

Sincerely,

Anita Bhattarai

www.ingramcontent.com/pod-product-compliance
Lightning Source LLC
Chambersburg PA
CBHW062100220526
45471CB00010B/3550